THE NEUROPSYCHIATRY OF CONSCIOUSNESS

THE NEUROPSYCHIATRY OF CONSCIOUSNESS

FRANCESCO MONACO
AND
ANDREA E. CAVANNA

Nova Biomedical Books

New York

LIBRARY OF CONGRESS CATALOGING-IN-PUBLICATION DATA

Monaco, Francesco.
The neuropsychiatry of consciousness / Francesco Monaco.
    p. ; cm.
Includes bibliographical references and index.
ISBN-13: 978-1-60021-860-6 (hardcover)
ISBN-10: 1-60021-860-1 (hardcover)
1. Consciousness--Physiological aspects.   2. Nervous system--Diseases--Pathophysiology.   3. Neuropsychiatry. I. Title.
    [DNLM: 1. Consciousness Disorders--physiopathology. 2. Consciousness--physiology. WL 341 M734n 2008]
    QP411.M58   2008
    612.8'2--dc22   2007030059

Published by Nova Science Publishers, Inc. ✦ New York

CONTENTS

Chapter 1   **Introduction**   **1**

1.1. Defining Consciousness   1

1.2. The Birth of Consciousness and The Case for Bicamerality   3

1.3. From Descartes to Philosophy of Mind   5

1.3.1. Renè Descartes: Mind-Body Dualism   5

1.3.2. David Chalmers: The Hard Problem   8

1.3.3. John Searle: The Emergent Consciousness   10

1.3.4. Daniel Dennett: Consciousness Explained (Away)   11

1.3.5. Paul Churchland: Eliminating Consciousness   12

1.3.6. Colin McGinn: The Mysterious Consciousness   14

1.4. References   16

Chapter 2   **In Search of the Neural Correlates of Consciousness**   **19**

2.1. The Neuroscience of Consciousness   19

2.2. Level and Contents of Consciousness   20

2.3. Consciousness Within the Neurosciences   22

2.3.1. John Eccles: Conscious Psychons   22

2.3.2. Francis Crick: The Astonishing Consciousness   24

2.3.3. Gerald Edelman: The Darwinian Consciousness   25

2.3.4. Antonio Damasio: Consciousness and Emotions   26

2.3.5. Bernard Baars: A Workspace For Consciousness   28

2.4. The Neuropsychiatry of Consciousness   29

2.5. References   30

Chapter 3   **Wakefulness and Sleep**   **35**

3.1. The Mysteries of Sleep   35

3.2. Regulation of The Sleep-Wake Cycle   36

3.2.1. Sleep Architecture   36

3.2.2. Neuroanatomical And Neurophysiological Bases of Sleep   41

3.2.3. Circadian Rhythms   43

3.3. Neurotransmitters of Sleep   44

3.4. The Genetic Regulation of Sleep   45

3.5. What Are Dreams Made of?   46
3.6. Pharmacological Modulation of Sleep   47
3.6.1. Psychostimulants And Wakefulness-Promoting Drugs   47
3.6.2. Hypnotics   49
3.7. The Neuroimaging of Sleep   52
3.8. Sleep Disorders   53
3.8.1. Hypersomnias   53
3.8.2. Sleep-Related Movement Disorders   54
3.9. Sleep And The Conscious Brain   55
3.10. References   56

Chapter 4   **Coma and Drug-Induced Anesthesia**   **61**
4.1. The Unresponsive Patient   61
4.2. What Causes Coma?   62
4.3. Coma – And Beyond   63
4.3.1. Brain Death   63
4.3.2. Coma   64
4.3.3. Vegetative State   64
4.3.4. Minimally Conscious State   65
4.3.5. Locked-in Syndrome   67
4.4. Imitators of Coma   67
4.5. The Assessment of The Unresponsive Patient   69
4.6. The Brain of The Unresponsive Patient   71
4.7. Drug-induced Anesthesia: Induction and Recovery   73
4.8. Functional Imaging of General Anesthesia   75
4.9. References   77

Chapter 5   **Transient Alterations of Consciousness: Epilepsy**   **85**
5.1. Epilepsy And Consciousness   85
5.2. Consciousness-affecting Seizures   86
5.3. Generalized Seizures as Transient Black-outs   87
5.4. Partial Seizures And Experiential Phenomena   89
5.4.1. Penfield's Experiments   91
5.4.2. The Neural Correlates of Epileptic Qualia   92
5.5. Limbic Status Epilepticus: The "Zombie State"   94
5.6. The Assessment of Consciousness in Temporal Lobe Epilepsy   96
5.7. A Window Over The Two Dimensions of Consciousness   98
5.8. References   99

Chapter 6   **Progressive Loss of Consciousness: Alzheimer's Disease**   **105**
6.1. When Consciousness Turns Off   105
6.2. Degenerative Dementias   107
6.2.1. Alzheimer's Disease   107
6.2.2. Pick's Disease   112
6.2.3. Frontotemporal Dementia   113
6.2.4. Movement Disorders Associated With Dementia   113

	6.3. Vascular Dementia	115
	6.4. Other Dementia Syndromes	116
	6.4.1. Normal Pressure Hydrocephalus	116
	6.4.2. Traumatic Dementia	116
	6.5. Mild Cognitive Impairment	117
	6.6. The Management of Dementia	117
	6.7. Reflective Consciousness in Patients With Dementia	119
	6.8. The Neurobiology of The Dwindling Self	119
	6.9. References	123
Chapter 7	**The Fragmented Self: Dissociative Disorders**	**129**
	7.1. Psychiatry And Consciousness	129
	7.2. Dissociative Amnesia	131
	7.3. Dissociative Fugue	131
	7.4. Depersonalization Disorder	132
	7.5. Dissociative Identity Disorder	133
	7.6. Hysteria	134
	7.7. The Neurobiology of Depersonalization	135
	7.8. The Neural Correlates of Dissociation	136
	7.9. Functional Neuroimaging of Conversion	138
	7.10. Consciousness in Psychoanalysis	138
	7.11. References	139
Chapter 8	**Conclusions: Mind, Matter, and the Conscious Brain**	**145**
Index		**149**

The nosology of insanity, the etiology, the symptomatology, pathology, diagnosis, prognosis, the care – how nicely the textbooks classified everything! How accurately they defined the idiot, the cretin, the imbecile, the epileptic, the hysteric, hypochondriac, and neurasthenic. Instead of admitting that little was known about what went on in the human brain, either healthy or sick, the professors stacked up Latin names.

I. Bashevis Singer, The Estate (1969)

I would like to dedicate this work to the patients who volunteered to endure hours of testing at our center. I have often learned more from my conversations with them, despite their damaged brains, than from my learned colleagues.

V. Ramachandran, Preface of BBC Reith Lectures (2003)

Chapter 1

INTRODUCTION
THE BORDERLANDS OF CONSCIOUSNESS

*Since the pineal gland is the only solid part in the whole brain which is single, it must
necessarily be the seat of the common sense, i.e. of thought, and consequently of the soul;
for one cannot be separated from the other.*
*The only alternative is to say that the soul is not joined immediately to any solid part of
the body, but only to the animal spirits which are in its concavities, and which enter it and
leave it continually like the water of river. That would certainly be thought too absurd.*

Renè Descartes, The Passions of the Soul (1649)

1.1. DEFINING CONSCIOUSNESS

Consciousness has been described as both the more obvious and the most mysterious
feature of our minds (Dennett 1987). On the one hand, there is nothing we know about more
directly than consciousness: what could be more certain or manifest to each of us than that he
or she is a subject of experience, an enjoyer of perceptions and sensations, a sufferer of pain,
an entertainer of ideas and a conscious deliberator? On the other hand, it is extraordinarily
hard to reconcile all these conscious experiences with everything else we know. What in the
world can consciousness be? How can physical bodies in the physical world contain such a
phenomenon? How could it possibly arise from neural processes in the brain? Science has
revealed the secrets of many initially mysterious natural phenomena – magnetism,
photosynthesis, digestion, reproduction – but consciousness seems utterly unlike these. Why?
Probably because particular cases of magnetism or photosynthesis or digestion are in
principle equally accessible to any observer with the right apparatus, but any particular case
of consciousness seems to have a favoured or privileged observer, whose access to the
phenomenon is entirely unlike, and better than, anyone else's, no matter what apparatus they
may have. For this reason and others, not only we have so far no good theory of

consciousness, we lack even a clear and uncontroversial pre-theoretical description of the presumed phenomenon.

Our view of the world is conditioned by the functioning of the brain. In this scientific era there is little to support the view that mind is more than neural networks and neurological processes. Science demands a neurocognitive explanation for all subjective experience. But here is the difficulty. For, as yet, we have no comprehensive scientific explanation of subjectivity. As Sherrington said, when using the energy scheme to trace the light from a star to the eye, retina, optic nerve, pathways and cortex: "At this point the scheme puts its finger in its lips and is silent". There is no explanation of how the star comes into subjective, conscious experience. It has been advocated that neuroscientists should take advantage of the conceptual tools provided by philosophers of mind (e.g. the concepts of mental representations and phenomenal states), since at least part of the difficulty encountered in tackling the problem of consciousness flows from the ambiguities of the term (Chalmers 1998; Churchland 1986; Churchland and Churchland 1997).

Consciousness has always defied any unequivocal definition. Attempts to define consciousness have yielded fairly different results over time (Markowitsch 1995; Searle 1997). Ancient philosophers generally ascribed consciousness to either the metaphysical concept of "being" or the religious notion of "soul". Things remained unchanged until the XVII century, when Descartes (1596-1650) restated the issue by theorizing a dualism between mind (so-called "res cogitans") and body ("res extensa") – see paragraph 3.1. The relationship connecting the two domains of reality was quite obscure and this mind-body split set up the mind-body problem as it is now conceived by folk psychology (Crane and Patterson 2000). Psychoanalytic theories have traditionally focused on the unconscious, rather than the conscious features of mind. During the first half of the last century, the doctrine of behaviorism rejected altogether the existence of any sort of mental ontology, in its effort to expel the "ghost" from of the "machine" (Ryle 1949). One of its main legacies is contemporary philosophical eliminativism about private mental states (Dennett 1991). In their landmark treatise of stupor and coma, Plum and Posner (1980) provided a tautological definition of consciousness as "awareness of self and the environment". Most neurophysiology textbooks define consciousness as a sum of cognitive functions, such as alertness, attention, perception, memory, and motivational systems (Bechtel and Graham 1998; Young 1998). In a recent and comprehensive review on consciousness, Zeman (2001) stressed the distinction between consciousness and self consciousness, and expanded both concepts: the former can be intended as "wakefulness", "experience", or "mind", while self-consciousness can convey five different meanings, encompassing "proneness to embarrassment", "self-detection", "self-recognition", "self-knowledge" and "awareness of awareness".

In sum, the search for a clear definition of consciousness appears to be never ending, as long as this term cuts across the domains of clinical medicine, neurosciences, psychology, and philosophy. As a matter of fact, the use of this concept varies according to the practical purpose of the investigation being conducted. In everyday clinical practice, consciousness is generally equated with the waking state, and the abilities to perceive, interact and communicate with the environment and with others in the integrated manner which wakefulness normally implies. The clinicians commonly use such terms as clouding, dwindling, waning, and lapsing of consciousness, meaning a reduced level of wakefulness and awareness (Fenwick 1994). Neurologists – and more specifically epileptologists – introduced the concept of "loss of contact" with the surrounding environment for a better description of the ictal conscious state (Gastaut 1970). Again, these terms are arguably useful in communicating the patient's responsiveness, but do little to further scientific understanding of conscious states as subjectively experienced by the patient.

This introductory chapter will encompass different ways of conceptualising the problem of consciousness and its relationship to an organic substrate (the brain), as provided by some of the leading thinkers and philosophers of mind (for a systematic approach the reader is referred to Flanagan 1992; Graham 1993; Guttenplan 1994; Kim 1996). The next section opens with some reflections on the evolutionary account of the appearance of consciousness in Homo sapiens.

1.2. THE BIRTH OF CONSCIOUSNESS AND THE CASE FOR BICAMERALITY

The issue of the development of a conscious mind from a phylogenetic perspective is one of the key topics of current philosophical and neuroscientific debate on consciousness. Can we say that Homo sapiens has always been experiencing consciousness of himself and others as we do now? Of course, to answer this question we need to look back into our past for evidence of metareflection – i.e. traces of self consciousness. A few years ago this issue has been addressed by a brilliant psychologist who adopted a multidisciplinary perspective. In our view, his pioneering work still stands as the best starting point for our brief journey in the field of consciousness studies.

In 1976 Julian Jaynes published his controversial book *The Origins of Consciousness in the Breakdown of the Bicameral Mind*, introducing the hypothesis of a two-chambered brain-mind model that preceded the evolutionary development of the conscious mind. Jaynes' speculative model of the bicameral mind, based on a wealth of archeological, anthropological, psychological, and neurological data (Jaynes 1976), gave rise to a huge debate, which has reverberated throughout the current neuroscientific and neurophilosophical literature (Cavanna et al. 2007). Not surprisingly, this thought-provoking and pioneering work in the field of consciousness studies gave rise to a longlasting debate, with contributions from a wide spectrum of disciplines (Dennett 1986; Jaynes 1986; Ojemann 1986). Even today, it has been argued that a multidisciplinary approach to the problem of consciousness and its development in the evolutionary process that shaped *Homo sapiens* cannot leave out an analysis of Jaynes' theory of the origin of consciousness in the breakdown of the preconscious bicameral mind (Donald 1991; Greenspan and Shanker 2004).

The background of Jaynes' evolutionary account of the transition from bicamerality to the conscious mind is the claim that human consciousness arises from the power of language to make metaphors and analogies. Metaphors of "me" and analogous models of "I" allow consciousness to function through introspection and self-visualization. According to this view, consciousness is a conceptual, metaphor-generated inner world that parallels the actual world and is intimately bound with volition and decision. *Homo sapiens*, therefore, could not experience consciousness until he developed a language sophisticated enough to produce metaphors and analogical models.

Jaynes recognizes that consciousness itself is only a small part of mental activity and is not necessary for sensation or perception, for concept formation, for learning, thinking or even reasoning. Thus, if major human actions and skills can function automatically and unconsciously, then it is conceivable that there were, at one time, human beings who did most of the things we do – speak, understand, perceive, solve problems – but who were without consciousness. Man's earliest writings (hieroglyphics, hieratic and cuneiform) are quite difficult for us to translate and understand in depth, especially when they refer to anything psychological. Thus, if we want to look for any historical evidence of consciousness – an analogous "I" narrating in a mind-space – we should go to a language with which we have some cultural continuity, and that is ancient Greek.

According to Jaynes, the earliest Greek text of sufficient size to test the question of whether there is any evidence of consciousness is the *Iliad*. In fact, the *Iliad* does not seem to mention any subjective thoughts or the contents of anyone's mind. The heroes of the *Iliad* were not able to make decisions, no one was introspecting or even reminiscing. Apparently, they were noble "automata" who were not aware of what they did. Iliadic man did not have subjectivity as we do; he had no internal mind-space to introspect upon.

It has been independently observed by a number of classical philologists (e.g. Onians 1951; Adkins 1970) that, unlike later writings, the Iliadic vocabulary lacks a single word for the concept of consciousness, or even mind (Taylor 1989). Instead, there exists a multitude of terms, referred to by Jaynes as "preconscious hypostases", that are thought to relate to physiological processes associated with mental life (Bremmer 1987). These "preconscious hypostases" are expressed by words like "psyche" (the living breath departing from the dead) (Darcus 1979), "thumos" (either the blowing breath or the flowing blood) (Caswell 1990), "phren" (almost always in the plural form "phrenes": presumably, the inflating lungs) (Darcus 1988), among others. Such lexical oddities apparently disappeared in subsequent milestones in Western literature, beginning with the *Odyssey*. The deep psychological analysis and the rich mental vocabulary that characterize Aeschylus' *Agamemnon* or Euripides' *Medea* (V-IV century B.C.), for instance, do not show any significant difference from what is found in most modern and contemporary literature. This is not the case for the composite text of the *Iliad*, which is peculiarly devoid of any psychological insight. As such, it stands out as a unique and unexplained model in Western culture (Taylor 1989). Similarly, it has been pointed out that in early Mycenaean figurative art, the human body was depicted as a curious aggregate of limbs, with marked joints and a fairly inconsistent trunk (Snell 1946; with a discussion in Feyerabend 1975). Greek classical art, on the other hand, closely resembled more recent figurative styles.

The lexical oddities detected in the Homeric text (especially the absence of a single word translating "consciousness", "mind", "soul", or even "body") led Jaynes to formulate the hypothesis that the *Iliad* was composed by nonconscious minds, which automatically recorded and objectively reported events, in a manner rather similar to the characters of the poem. The transition to subjective and introspective writings of the conscious mind occurred in later times, beginning with the *Odyssey*.

In short, Jaynes claimed that men in the age of the *Iliad* learned to speak, read, write, as well as conduct their daily lives, yet remained nonconscious throughout their lives. Being nonconscious, they were not responsible for their actions. Who, then, made the decisions? Jaynes' answer was that whenever a significant choice was to be made, an auditory hallucination intervened, telling people what to do. These voices, in the *Iliad* always and immediately obeyed, were called Gods. Before the cultural evolution of consciousness, the human brain was organized in a bicameral fashion: the right hemisphere (the synthetic, poetic, "god-brain") used to transmit hallucinatory verbal instructions to the left hemisphere (the analytical, rational, "man-brain"), especially in response to unusual or stressful situations. It follows that human mentality was divided into two parts, a decision-making part (located in the right hemisphere) and a follower part (in the left hemisphere), and neither part was "conscious". According to Jaynes, the bicameral mind is to be observed not only in the most ancient literature but also in the contemporary examples of throwbacks to bicamerality, such as hypnosis and schizophrenia, since auditory or verbal hallucinations can be regarded as a remnant of this early mentality. Moreover, the bicameral mentality allowed a large group to carry around with them, in the form of verbal hallucinations, the directions of the king. The leaders used these stress-generated "voices" to lead the masses in cooperative unison. The bicameral mind enabled men to build societies and the earliest civilizations (the Near East, Egypt, Southern Africa, India, China, Mesoamerica), developed through common hallucinating voices attributed to Gods and other rulers – i.e. external "authorities" – and to various symbols, such as graves, temples, and idols.

Finally, Jaynes speculated that the development of modern human consciousness began as late as around 1400-600 B.C., when men were evolutionarily forced by the chaos of huge migrations induced by overpopulation and natural catastrophes, and by the widespread use of writing, to change their mentality.

While innovative and thought-provoking, Jaynes' sophisticated hypothesis presents with several difficulties, as shown by the criticism it attracted from different angles (for a recent review, see Cavanna et al. 2007). Moreover, recent neurobiological and neurophysiological data provide weak support for a bicameral structure of the preconscious mind (e.g. Sher 2000). However there is little doubt that significant paradigm shifts regarding the concept of consciousness took place in ancient times, as documented in literary texts. Adopting the brain-computer analogy, Jaynes' theory stands out as a very interesting account for some software (=cultural), rather than hardware (=structural), developments of the brain/mind continuum (Dennett 1986).

1.3. FROM DESCARTES TO PHILOSOPHY OF MIND

1.3.1. Renè Descartes: Mind-Body Dualism

Modern philosophy of mind was born when French philosopher René Descartes (1596-1650) first addressed the question of the relationship between consciousness and brain by referring to the dualism of mind and matter ("Cartesian cut") (Atmanspacher 1994). Descartes' philosophical writings are very rich and cover much more than the split of matter and mind (Cottingham et al. 1984). He was a pure rationalist and developed the idea that we must distinguish two kind of substances only by logical reasoning. The method he used to base the existence of these two substances is well known (Watson 2002). He started by asking himself what he could take for real, and realised that everything could be unreal except his faculty of thinking. Things and sensations can be mere illusions, but a mind that, for instance, sees objects and listens to sounds – even though these objects and sounds are fictitious – must necessarily exist. Descartes calls his thinking "res cogitans", as opposed to the "res extensa". In Descartes' terminology, the entire reality consists of a material component ("res extensa") and a non-material component ("res cogitans"): literally translated, these labels characterize the realms of "extended substance" and "thinking substance". The notion of extension in "res extensa" means that the material reality is extended in its spatial location and in its temporal duration. The notion of cognition in "res cogitans" is probably best explained by referring to conscious activity in general rather than "thinking" in the narrow sense of intellectual capability. Interestingly enough, Descartes does not clearly distinguish the unconscious stream of thought from the conscious one. According to the French philosopher, "thinking" always means "thinking consciously".

Therefore, the Cartesian cut can be regarded as a conceptual border between matter and mind: these two realms can be denoted in many different ways, including the brain-mind dichotomy, all of which however represent variations of the radically dualistic scheme based on the definite distinction of the two substances. Descartes explicitly expressed the criterion for determining whether a function belongs to the body or the soul: "Anything we experience as being in us, and which we see can also exist in wholly inanimate bodies, must be attributed only to our body. On the other hand, anything in us which we cannot conceive in any way as capable of belonging to a body must be attributed to our soul. Thus, because we have no conception of the body as thinking in any way at all, we have reason to believe that every kind of thought present in us belongs to the soul. And since we do not doubt that there are inanimate bodies which can move in as many different ways as our bodies, if not more, and which have as much heat or more […], we must believe that all the heat and all the movements present in us, in so far as they do not depend on thought, belong solely to the body" (Cottingham et al. 1984).

Descartes was a dualistic interactionist, who thought that the rational soul and the body have a causal influence on each other. Obviously, the main problem with this view was to give an account of how mind and matter could interact. Descartes' solution was to find out, first of all, the place where such interaction could occur, and then to try to understand its functioning. *Les passions de l'ame* (1649) (Figure 1.1) represents Descartes' most important contribution to psychology proper and overall consciousness studies.

In addition to an analysis of primary emotions, it contains Descartes' most extensive account of causal mind/body interactionism and of the localization of the soul's contact with the body in the pineal gland. He chose this gland because it appeared to be the only organ in the brain that was not bilaterally duplicated and because he believed, erroneously, that it was uniquely human. "My view is that this gland is the principal seat of the soul – he wrote – and the place in which all our thoughts are formed. The reason I believe this is that I cannot find any part of the brain, except this, which is not double. Since we see only one thing with two eyes, and hear only one voice with two ears, and in short have never more than one thought at a time, it must necessarily be the case that the impressions which enter by the two eyes or by the two ears, and so on, unite with each other in some part of the body before being considered by the soul. Now it is impossible to find any such place in the whole head except this gland; moreover it is situated in the most suitable possible place for this purpose, in the middle of all the concavities; and it is supported and surrounded by the little branches of the carotid arteries which bring the spirits into the brain" (Cottingham et al. 1984). According to Descartes, all intellectual properties have their seat in the pineal gland, including the *sensus communis*, the general faculty of sense. The pineal gland was the place where the "res cogitans" and the "res extensa" met together. Through this organ, the soul is joined to the body in a way that forms a functional unit (Cottingham et al. 1984).

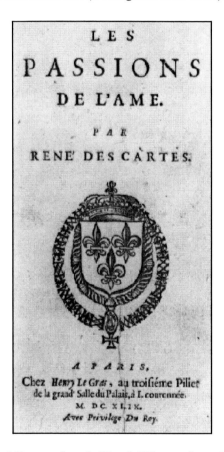

Figure 1.1. Cover of Descartes' "Les passions de l'âme" ("The passions of the soul") 1649.

Only a few people accepted Descartes' pineal neurophysiology when he was still alive, and it was almost universally rejected after his death. Willis wrote about the pineal gland that "we can scarce believe this to be the seat of the Soul, or its chief Faculties to arise from it; because Animals, which seem to be almost quite destitute of Imagination, Memory, and other superior Powers of the Soul, have this Glandula or Kernel large and fair enough" (Willis 1681). Other critics undermined the very idea of interaction itself. According to them, it is not possible for the soul and the body to have a causal influence on each other since the mind, having no extension, no mass, no force fields – in sum, no physical properties at all – could not have a chance to cause the slightest change in the physical realm.

Despite the criticism it attracted, Cartesian dualism is of central importance for the worldview that Western science and philosophy have developed. On the other hand, it is obvious that the distinction it makes is nothing more than a conceptual tool and should be taken seriously at the level of abstraction, where both its origin and its power lie. Since consciousness represents a non-material object within "res cogitans", theoretically it could not possibly be studied as an object of physics in the conventional sense.

1.3.2. David Chalmers: The Hard Problem

In order to clarify the issue of consciousness, contemporary American philosopher David Chalmers clearly separated the problems that are often clustered together under the same name. For this purpose, he distinguished between the "easy problems" and the "hard problem" of consciousness (Chalmers 1996).

The easy problems of consciousness include the following issues: How can we discriminate sensory stimuli and react to them appropriately? How does the brain integrate information from different sources and use this information to control purposeful behavior? How is it that subjects can verbalize their internal states? Although all these questions are associated with consciousness, they basically concern the objective mechanisms of the cognitive system. Consequently, we can reasonably expect that continued work in cognitive psychology and neuroscience will find proper answers to them.

On the other hand, the hard problem is the question of how physical processes occurring in the brain give rise to subjective experience at all. This puzzle involves the inner aspect of thought and perception: the way things feel for the subject. When we see a red object, for example, we experience visual sensations, such as that of vivid "redness". The same happens when we hear the ineffable sound of a violin, when we feel the agony of an intense pain, and so forth. Within these phenomena Chalmers poses the real mystery of the mind.

Needless to say, the easy problems are by no means trivial - they are actually as challenging as most in psychology and neurobiology - however it is with the hard problem that we have to deal if we want to provide a scientifically sound account of our everyday conscious experiences (Chalmers 2000).

The distinction between the easy problems and the hard problem is well illustrated by a widely quoted thought experiment devised by an Australian philosopher, Frank Jackson (1982). Suppose that Mary, a neuroscientist living in the 23rd century, is the world's leading expert on the brain processes responsible for color vision. Unfortunately, Mary has lived her whole life in a black-and-white room and has never seen any other colors. Therefore, she is in the following situation: she knows everything there is to know about physical processes in the brain subserving color vision. This understanding enables her to grasp all there is to know about the easy problems: how the brain discriminates stimuli, integrates information and produces verbal reports. She is expected to know how color names correspond with wavelengths on the light spectrum. But there is still something crucial about color vision that Mary does not know: what it is like to experience a color such as red. This thought experiment argues that there are facts about conscious experience that cannot be deduced from knowledge about the physical functioning of the brain.

These private facts are sometimes referred to as subjective, "phenomenal" experiences - or "*qualia*", according to the philosophical jargon (Nagel 1979) recently translated into the neuroscientific lexicon (e.g. Monaco et al. 2005). Philosophers of mind use this technical term to refer to the subjective texture of experience, which is the essence of the qualitative dimension of consciousness. Roughly speaking, a quale (singular of qualia) is the "what it is like" character of mental states: the way it feels to have mental states such as pain, seeing red, smelling a rose, etc. Therefore, qualia are experiential properties of sensations, feelings, perceptions and, more controversially, thoughts and desires (Block 2004). The status of qualia is hotly debated in both philosophy and neuroscience, largely because it stays at the heart of the hard problem and is central to a proper understanding of the nature of consciousness (Gray 2003). Qualia are by definition subjective entities: I can not be sure that another person's "red" is identical to my red. Whereas science offers us a third-person view of the world, qualia offers only what appears to be a first-person view. I have a privileged perspective on what it feels like to be me that is not available to anyone else: someone else may sympathize with my feelings, joys and sorrows, but only *I* can actually experience them. Even if we accept that mental states are the product of brain-states, at present it is not possible for the neuroscientist to peer inside my brain and see what I am feeling. Indeed, we routinely hide our inner world from others. Such intrinsic 'first-person' aspect of consciousness makes it difficult to assimilate into the scientific world-picture, since science deals with what is observable and measurable and consciousness arguably conforms to none of these requirements. Though this problem has loomed large recently, it is not a new problem. Charles Darwin (1809-1892), the greatest biologist of all times and the designer of the theory of the evolution of species by natural selection, pondered on this problem - or something very like it - in his notebooks. In the final analysis he seemed as baffled as anyone else and resigned to the fact that our knowledge of matter is quite insufficient to account for the phenomena [the conscious appearance] of thought, and referred to the origin of consciousness as 'mysterious'. Biologist Thomas Henry Huxley (1825-1895), who vigorously championed Darwin's theory of evolution against the objections from both the clergy and the scientific community of the time, expressed this same bafflement using a celebrated metaphor:

"*We class sensations along with emotions, and volitions, and thoughts, under the common head of states of consciousness. But what consciousness is, we know not; and how it is that anything so remarkable as a state of consciousness comes about as the result of irritating nervous tissue, is just as unaccountable as the appearance of the Djin when Aladdin rubbed his lamp in the story, or as any other ultimate fact of nature.*"

Likewise, Chalmers argues that consciousness cannot be explained by adopting a reductionist approach, because it does not belong to the realm of matter (Chalmers 1996; 1998). He proposes to expand science in a fashion that is still compatible with a dualist approach. Chalmers' ontology admits both physical and non-physical features in the world. His dualism is different from Descartes' in that it claims that "consciousness is a feature of the world" which is somehow related to its physical properties. Chalmers offers an interpretation of his theory based on the dualism between "information" and "pattern": within this conceptual framework, consciousness is information about the pattern of the self. Information becomes therefore the link between the physical and the conscious. Ultimately, and quite similarly to the philosophical doctrine of panpsychism, everything having these properties may be conscious, at least to some degree.

1.3.3. John Searle: The Emergent Consciousness

According to philosopher of mind John Searle, the most important scientific discovery of the present era will come when someone finds the answer to the following question: how exactly do neurobiological processes in the brain cause consciousness? This is the most important question faced by the biological sciences, and yet it is frequently evaded or misunderstood (Searle 1998). Searle claims that this question mirrors the (in)famous "mind-body problem" which has a long and controversial history in both philosophy and science. He thinks that the mind-body problem has a rather simple solution: conscious states are caused by lower level neurobiological processes in the brain and are themselves higher level features of the brain (Searle 1992; 2004).

However, a crucial question remains: what is the form of existence of these conscious processes? More pointedly, does the claim that there is a causal relation between brain and consciousness commit us to an ontological dualism of "physical" things and "mental" things? Searle's answer is a definite no. Brain processes cause consciousness but the consciousness they cause is not some extra substance or entity. It is just a higher level feature of the brain system. The two crucial relationships between consciousness and the brain, then, can be summarized as follows: lower-level neuronal processes in the brain cause consciousness and consciousness is simply a higher-level feature of the system that is made up of the lower-level neuronal elements (Searle 1997).

Searle quotes several examples in nature where a higher-level feature of a system is caused by lower-level elements, even though the feature is made up of those elements. Such examples include the liquidity of water, the transparency of glass, the solidity of a table, and so forth. According to these analogies, The experience of "redness" while seeing a rose occur at a much higher level than that of the single neuron or synapse, just as liquidity occurs at a much higher level than that of single molecules. However, there is no metaphysical or logical obstacle to claiming that the relationship between brain and consciousness is one of causation and at the same time claiming that consciousness is just a feature of the brain.

Searle argues that we simply know as a matter of fact that brain processes cause conscious states. We do not know the details about how it works and it may well be a long time before we fully understand it. Furthermore, he suggests that an understanding of how exactly brain processes cause conscious states may require a revolution in neurobiology. It is not at all obvious how, within our present explanatory apparatus, we can account for the causal character of the relationship between neuron firings and conscious states. But, at present, from the fact that we do not know *how* it occurs, it does not follow that we do not know *that* it occurs. The problem of how exactly the brain system works to produce consciousness is an empirical/theoretical issue for the neurobiological sciences (Searle 1997).

The central role of neurobiological processes for the emergence of consciousness reflects Searle's arguments against the project of Artificial Intelligence that sees the mind as a sort of computer (Searle 1990). In a paper which first appeared in 1980 and has never been out of print since, Searle put forward the famous 'Chinese Room' argument. Briefly, this thought experiment is the story of a man sitting in a room with a big manual full of symbols. From time to time, someone slides a card with some symbols on it into the room through a slot in the wall. The man in the room looks up the symbols in his book, and in accordance with its instructions selects another card with symbols on and pushes it out through the slot. The symbols are in fact Chinese characters, and it appears to the person outside the room that he is having a conversation in Chinese with the man in the room. The question is: does this show that the man in the room understands Chinese? For Searle, the obvious answer is no. There is a difference between running a computer program (to which this thought-experiment is an analogy) and having conscious knowledge. The computer operates by manipulating symbols, but only the human brain attaches meaning to those symbols. It is a fact of the matter that neurobiological processes produce conscious mental phenomena that are irreducibly subjective. Searle's conclusion leaves no hope for the most ambitious project of Artificial Intelligence: machines will never be able to reproduce human consciousness, because it seems that consciousness spontaneously emerges in presence of determined natural conditions that can not be artificially recreated.

1.3.4. Daniel Dennett: Consciousness Explained (Away)

The influential American philosopher Daniel Dennett is one of the pioneers in the field of consciousness studies: his first book on the subject, *Content and Consciousness,* appeared back in 1969, and he has continued to refine and build his views in a long series of papers and books (e.g. Dennett 1978; 1991; 2001; 2005). Dennett advocates a third-person approach to consciousness (what he calls "heterophenomenology") - that is, we try to investigate the contents of consciousness from the outside to the point where we can claim that what we have discovered is 'without significant residue'. Heterophenomenology shows that, despite the apparent unity and continuity of our experience, consciousness does not involve the existence of a single central self. Instead, according to Dennett, the mind is occupied by several parallel "drafts". A "draft" can be roughly viewed as a narrative that occurs in the mind, and that is typically triggered by some interaction with the external environment. At every point in time, one of those narratives is dominant in the brain, and that is what we are conscious of. As a consequence, "consciousness" is a vague term which simply refers to the feeling of the overall brain activity. But the truth is that there are many drafts, all working in parallel, and there are several narratives in the mind going on at the same time. A mental content becomes conscious by winning the competition with other mental contents and therefore lasting longer in the mind. Consciousness is nothing more than an organization of competing mental events. It is undeniable that Dennett, in attempting to make consciousness less mysterious, is also trying to chip away at what we think of as our intrinsically subjective experiences or 'qualia'. Basically, Dennett claims that qualia, and conscious states in general, do not exist in the way we think of them (Dennett 1988).

It has been claimed that Dennett not so much explains consciousness as attempts to explain it away. More precisely, what Dennett he is trying to do is to show that consciousness is not what we have taken it to be. For Dennett, it is not the case that we are the privileged observers of our own mental states. We are simply not authoritative about what is happening in our heads, but only about what *seems* to be happening in our heads. For instance, often we are not conscious of what is happening inside us until somebody else asks about it. According to the principle that "probing precipitates narratives", it may be only when pointed out to us how we are behaving towards that person that we become aware of our feelings and – perhaps reluctantly – admit to them. Experiments with subjects who are put under hypnosis have provided compelling evidence for this. Dennett holds, in effect, that we are always telling stories to ourselves. Certainly, consciousness is an emergent property from a complex organization of physical systems but, as he points out, although different parts of the brain have been shown to be associated with different sorts of mental activity, there is no part of the brain that serves to co-ordinate or direct all those sub-activities. Using Dennett's words, there is no "Cartesian theatre" (a centered locus in the brain that directs consciousness), where all varieties of perceptions and thoughts are accomplished by parallel, multitrack brain processes. Rather, on his model there is pandemonium - lots of small agents (called "homunculi") competing for attention with no central headquarters in control. We must think of multiple channels exerting simultaneous influence, of a variety of cognitive sub-systems talking to one another. None of these is, strictly speaking, conscious, and the brain is not different from a sophisticated computer that runs parallel, multitrack processes.

1.3.5. Paul Churchland: Eliminating Consciousness

Canadian philosopher Paul Churchland develops Dennett's stance to its extreme consequences by arguing that our commonsense concept of consciousness and other psychological phenomena is a radically false theory in the way that talk about demons as the cause of epilepsy or talk about phlogiston as the cause of combustibility, are radically false theories (Churchland 1985; 1995). Churchland (1981) uncompromisingly advocates the damnation of mental discourse and all its works in all contexts. Our ordinary mental descriptions are usually described by him as our "folk psychology". This is, of course, a pejorative term, as it immediately calls to mind "folk medicine" or "folk science". To get a witch-doctor or a quack to treat epilepsy by exorcism is not merely to act on a false theory, it is to put the patient in mortal danger. In a similar fashion, we should think of "folk psychology" as not only false but also potentially dangerous.

Churchland's idea is that in future all those common psychological concepts – which in analytical philosophy are best known as "propositional attitudes" – will be replaced by chemical patterns, physical structures and neurobiological categories. Contrary to the commonsense view, Churchland claims that our propositional attitudes or feelings and emotions are wholly reducible to precise physical states, events or processes occurring in our brains. This means that we are nothing more than an extremely well organized pattern of neural networks.

Overall, Churchland's eliminativism is based on a strong belief in the reductionistic approach (Churchland and Churchland 1990). Theoretically, we should be able to give a neurophysiological account for what happens when, for instance, we are worried about a friend or when we are feeling uneasy because we have to speak at a conference. According to this view, the mind-body problem is nothing but a pseudo-problem: we have to deal with the same phenomenon observed from different perspectives, as happened in astronomy when we discovered that the Morning Star and the Evening Star were exactly the same entity (i.e. the planet Venus). Likewise, we will find out that propositions having mental vocabulary and propositions having solely physical vocabulary basically refer to the same phenomena. The difference between the two kinds of propositions is due to a mere change of perspective. Hence, saying that a human being is in pain is equivalent to saying that his C-fibres are excited so-and-so, with the little difference that speaking of pain means to give a first-person account of the fact – i.e. an account given by who actually is in that situation – whereas speaking of another person's C-fibres excitement means to give a third-person account of the same fact – i.e. an account given by the observer of another person's C-fibres excited so-and-so.

The only true distinction between the two vocabularies pertains to their linguistic forms: the accounts reported in the first-person perspective are somewhat equivocal and confused, whereas the accounts reported in the third-person perspective are more precise and clear. Nevertheless, they have no *substantial* difference. According to Churchland, there is nothing more in the direct experience of pain that can not be expressed in neurophysiological vocabulary (Churchland and Churchland 1990; 1997).

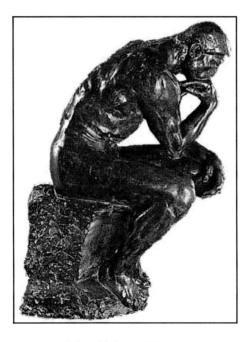

Figure 1.2. Auguste Rodin, *Le Penseur* (The Thinker), 1880.

Seen against the background of twentieth century philosophy, eliminative materialism could be seen as the apotheosis of the logical positivist programme of translating mental descriptions into physical ones. In effect, Churchland advocates something even stronger, namely the bypassing of any work of translation in favor of the complete elimination or liquidation of mental descriptions. With this liquidation of even any mention of mental states or events, eliminative materialism aims at performing a sort of philosophical 'disappearance trick' with the so-called "problem of privacy" i.e. the problem of giving a scientifically sound account for first-person (subjective) experiences. If Churchland's perspective is right, when Rodin's *Le Penseur* (Figure 1.2) is sitting in contemplation upon his rock, all that is going on, and so all we should ever talk about, are neurophysiological processes, and neurophysiologists are increasingly able and willing to tell us about them (Lyons 2001).

1.3.6. Colin McGinn: The Mysterious Consciousness

The British philosopher Colin McGinn is rather skeptical about the role of the neuroscientists in dissolving the mysteries that surround consciousness: for him the mere discovery of further empirical correlations between the mental and the physical is never going to bring the two conceptually together (McGinn 2004). It is not enough to assert, as Searle and others do, that some physical states give rise to mental states: we need an explanation of why some do so and others do not. McGinn quotes Saul Kripke's claim that when God created pain he had to do more than create C-fibre firing, whereas to create heat it sufficed to create molecular motion. That is to say, heat reduces without residue to molecular motion, but pain can never be reduced without residue to events in the brain. McGinn then goes on to question the feasibility of arriving at a coherent account as to how this is possible, thus attracting the label of 'Mysterian'. In fact, he accepts that there is a naturalistic explanation of how physical processes can give rise to mental ones, only he doubts that we as human beings are capable of arriving at that explanation (McGinn 2004).

McGinn claims that consciousness cannot be understood by beings with minds like ours. Inspired part by Russell and part by Kant, McGinn thinks that consciousness is known by the faculty of introspection, as opposed to the physical world, which is known by the faculty of perception. By asking if our cognitive closure is infinite, McGinn wonders if there is something in the world that we can not understand. His answer is that our cognitive closure is not infinite, that there are things we will never be capable of understanding - and consciousness is one of them. As he puts in, "mind may just not be big enough to understand mind".

In Aristotelian terms, the relationship between consciousness and brain is "noumenal", or impossible to understand: it is provided by a lower level of consciousness which is not accessible to introspection. In other words, understanding our consciousness is beyond our cognitive capacities, just like a child cannot grasp complex abstract concepts. McGinn notices that other creatures in nature lack the capability to understand things that we understand (e.g. the general theory of relativity). Since we are also creatures of nature, there is no reason to exclude that we also lack the capability of understanding something of nature.

Some of the best minds from the ancient Greeks to the present day have grappled with a series of problems - such as that of free will, of the nature of the self, the question of *a priori* and empirical knowledge - and still not come up with generally acceptable solutions. This is not because of any lack of intelligence in the philosophers concerned but rather because such problems are, in McGinn's words, "beyond the rim of human intellectual competence". That such problems are found to be intractable is not to suggest that they are meaningless or that there is no answer, only that the answer is, because of the way natural selection has built our brains, simply not available to us.

The American philosopher Thomas Nagel (1979) pointed out that we can only conceive of things as they appear to us and never as they are in themselves. We can only experience how it feels to be ourselves. We can never experience how it feels to be something else, for the simple reason that we are not something else. As Nagel wrote in a famous paper, we can learn all about the brain mechanisms of a bat's sonar system but we will never have the slightest idea of what it is like to have the sonar experiences of a bat ("what it is like to be a bat").

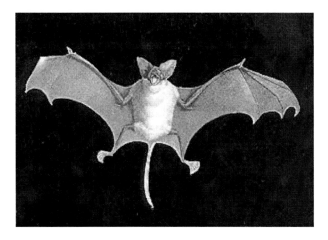

Figure 1.3. According to Thomas Nagel's mental experiment, nobody is able to experience "what it is like to be a bat", e.g. what it feels like gaining spatial information by means of ultrasounds, as bats do.

As in Frank Jackson's experiment on the color-blind neuroscientist (see paragraph 3.2), understanding how the brain works may not be enough to understand consciousness. Indeed, McGinn may be right that there are necessary limits to human knowledge, but one of those limits may well be that we can never discover where those limits lie. McGinn's project is essentially a Kantian one. Immanuel Kant once decreed that human understanding was such that we necessarily saw the world in terms of cause and effect, and in terms of Euclidean space. As we now know, he was wrong on both these counts, though he could scarcely have foreseen quantum physics or relativity theory. It is premature to say that McGinn has won the day, and it is likely that philosophers and neuroscientists will continue to battle on for a good while yet.

1.4. REFERENCES

Adkins ADH. *From the Many to the One: a Study of Personality and Views of Human Nature in the Context of Ancient Greek Society, Values and Beliefs.* Ithaca, NY; Cornell University Press 1970.

Atmanspacher H. Complexity, meaning and the Cartesian cut. *J Consciousness Studies* 1994;1:168-181.

Bechtel W, Graham G (Eds). *A companion to cognitive science.* Oxford, UK: Blackwell 1998.

Block N. Qualia. In: Gregory R, ed. *The Oxford Companion to the Mind.* Oxford; Oxford University Press 2004: 785-789.

Bremmer J. *The Early Greek Concept of the Soul. Princeton*; Princeton University Press 1987.

Caswell C. *A Study of Thumos in Early-Greek Epic.* Leiden; Brill 1990.

Cavanna AE, Trimble MR, Cinti F, Monaco F. The "bicameral mind" 30 years on: a critical reappraisal of Julian Jaynes' hypothesis. *Funct Neurol.* 2007;22:11-15.

Chalmers D. *The conscious mind: in search of a fundamental theory.* Oxford: Oxford University Press 1996.

Chalmers D. The problems of consciousness. *Adv Neurol.* 1998;77:7-18.

Chalmers D. What is a neural correlate of consciousness? In: Metzinger T, ed. *Neural correlates of consciousness: empirical and conceptual questions* MIT Press 2000;17-40.

Churchland P. Eliminative Materialism and the Propositional Attitudes. *J Philosophy* 1981;78:67-90.

Churchland PM, Churchland PS. Intertheoretic reduction: a neuroscientist's field guide. *Semin Neurosci* 1990;2:249-256.

Churchland PM, Churchland PS. Recent work on consciousness: philosophical, theoretical, and empirical. *Semin Neurol* 1997;17:179-186.

Churchland PM. *Matter and consciousness.* Cambridge, MA: MIT Press 1985.

Churchland PM. *The engine of reason, the seat of the soul: a philosophical journey into the brain.* Cambridge, MA: MIT Press 1995.

Churchland PS. *Neurophilosophy.* Cambridge, MA: MIT Press; 1986.

Cottingham J, Stoothoff R, Murdoch D. *The Philosophical Writings of Descartes.* Cambridge: Cambridge University Press 1984.

Crane T, Patterson S (Eds). *History of the mind-body problem.* New York, NY: Routledge 2000.

Darcus S. *A person's relation to psyche in Homer, Hesiod and Greek lyric poets.* Glotta 1979; 67: 30-39.

Darcus S. *Psychological Activity in Homer. A Study of Phren. Ottawa*; Carleton University Press 1988.

Dennett DC. Are we explaining consciousness yet? *Cognition* 2001;79:221-237.

Dennett DC. *Consciousness explained.* Boston, MA: Little, Brown 1991.

Dennett DC. *Quining qualia.* In: Marcel AJ, Bisiach E (eds) Consciousness in contemporary science Oxford: Clarendon Press 1988; 42-77.

Dennett DC. *Sweet Dreams: Philosophical Obstacles to a Science of Consciousness.* Cambridge, MA: MIT Press 2005.

Dennett DC. *Brainstorms.* Montgomery, Vermont: Bradford Books 1978.

Dennett DC. *Consciousness.* In: Gregory RL (ed) *The Oxford companion to the mind.* Oxford: Oxford University Press 1987. p. 160-164.

Dennett DC. Julian Jaynes' software archeology. *Canadian Psychology* 1986; 27:149-154.

Descartes R. *Les passions de l'âme.* Amsterdam: Elsevier 1649.

Donald M. *Origins of the Modern Mind: Three Stages in the Evolution of Culture and Cognition.* Cambridge, MA: Harvard University Press 1991.

Fenwick P, Alterations in conscious awareness. In Critchley EMR (Ed) *The neurological boundaries of reality.* London: Farrand Press 1994, p. 121-142.

Feyerabend PK. *Against Method: Outline of an Anarchistic Theory of Knowledge.* London; Verso 1975.

Flanagan O. *The science of the mind.* Cambridge, MA: MIT Press 1992.

Gastaut H. Clinical and electroencephalographical classification of epileptic seizures. *Epilepsia* 1970;11:102-113.

Graham G. *Philosophy of mind: an introduction.* Oxford, UK: Blackwell 1993.

Gray J. How are qualia coupled to functions? *Trends Cogn Sci.* 2003;7:192-194.

Greenspan SI, Shanker SG. *The First Idea: How Symbols, Language, and Intelligence Evolved from our Primate Ancestors to Modern Humans.* Cambridge, MA: DaCapo Press 2004.

Guttenplan S (Ed). *A companion to the philosophy of mind.* Oxford, UK: Blackwell 1994.

Jackson F. Epiphenomenal qualia. *Philosophical Quarterly.* 1982;32:127-136.

Jaynes J. Consciousness and the voices of the mind. *Canadian Psychology* 1986; 27:128-139.

Jaynes J. *The Origins of Consciousness in the Breakdown of the Bicameral Mind.* Boston, MA: Houghton Mifflin 1976.

Kim J. *Philosophy of mind.* Boulder, CO: Westview Press 1996.

Lyons W. *Matters of the mind.* Edinburgh: Edinburgh University Press 2001.

Markowitsch HJ. Cerebral basis of consciousness: a historical review. *Neuropsychologia* 1995;33:1181-1192.

McGinn C. *The mysterious flame: conscious minds in a material world.* New York: Basic Books 1999.

McGinn C. *Consciousness and its Objects.* Oxford: Oxford University Press 2004.

Monaco F, Mula M, Cavanna AE. Consciousness, epilepsy and emotional qualia. *Epilepsy Behav.* 2005;7:150-160.

Nagel T. What is it like to be a bat? In: *Mortal Questions.* Cambridge; Cambridge University Press 1979:165-180.

Ojemann G. Brain mechanisms for consciousness and conscious experience. *Canadian Psychology* 1986; 27:158-168.

Onians R. *The Origins of European Thought about the Body, the Mind, the Soul, the World, Time and Fate.* Cambridge; Cambridge University Press 1951.

Plum F, Posner JB. *The diagnosis of stupor and coma.* Philadelphia: Davis; 1980.

Ryle G. *The concept of mind.* New York: Barnes and Noble; 1949.

Searle J. How to study consciousness scientifically. *Philos Trans R Soc Lond B Biol Sci* 1998;353:1935-42.

Searle J. *Mind: A Brief Introduction* Oxford: Oxford University Press 2004.

Searle J. *The mystery of consciousness.* London: Granta Book 1997.

Searle J. *The rediscovery of the mind.* Cambridge, MA: MIT Press 1992.

Searle J. *Who is computing with the brain?* Behav Brain Sci 1990;13:632-42.

Sher L. Neuroimaging, auditory hallucinations, and the bicameral mind. *J Psychiatry Neurosci* 2000; 25:239-240.

Snell B. *Die Entdeckung des Geistes. Studien zur Entstehung des Europaischen Denkens bei den Griechen.* Hamburg; Claassen Verlag 1946.

Taylor C. *Sources of the Self.* Cambridge; Cambridge University Press 1989.

Watson R. *Cogito Ergo Sum: The Life of René Descartes*, Boston: Godine 2002.

Willis T. The anatomy of the brain and the description and use of the nerves. In: *The Remaining Medical Works of That Famous and Renowned Physician Dr. Thomas Willis*, translated by S. Pordage, London: Dring 1681.

Young GB. Consciousness. In: Young GB, Ropper AH, Bolton CF, editors. *Coma and impaired consciousness*. New York: McGraw-Hill; 1998. p.3-37.

Zeman A. Consciousness. *Brain* 2001;124:1263-1289.

IN SEARCH OF THE NEURAL CORRELATES OF CONSCIOUSNESS

*THE DEVIL. You conclude, then, that Life
was driving at clumsiness and ugliness?*

*DON JUAN. No, perverse devil that you are,
a thousand times no. Life was driving at brains –
at its darling object: an organ by which it can attain
not only self-consciousness but self-understanding.*

G.B. Shaw, Man and Superman, Act III (1903)

2.1. THE NEUROSCIENCE OF CONSCIOUSNESS

From being a neglected aspect of the philosophy of mind the problem of consciousness
has moved in recent years to be one of the hottest topics of neuroscientific debate. Much
progress has been made in the investigation of the neural correlates of consciousness;
however neuroscientific theories are far from reaching a consensus. Interestingly enough, all
these theories are scientifically sound, experimentally grounded, and start from what is
essentially the same standpoint, that of scientific naturalism. That is, all believe that human
consciousness is dependent on brain states, and that it has emerged by Darwinian
mechanisms as a natural (rather than supernatural) feature of the world. But that is where the
consensus ends.

Over the last decade there has been a heightened interest in attacking the problem of
consciousness through scientific investigation (Flanagan 1995; Searle 1998; Zeman 2003;
Koch 2004). A growing literature now tackles the issue of consciousness from a
neuroscientific perspective, as it has seemingly been transferred from philosophical debate to
empirical scrutiny. Newly instituted journals, associations and meetings are entirely devoted
to the scientific study of consciousness and related phenomena. The problem of

consciousness is largely debated across disciplines ranging across basic neuroscience, neurology, and psychiatry. The main issue is generally thought to be the explanation of how brain processes cause consciousness and how consciousness is realized in the brain (Crick and Koch 1998; Searle 2000).

In spite of the remarkably different perspectives of empirical and theoretical research, most of the disciplines found a common agreement about some kind of psychophysical correlation between mental and brain states: every mental state (state of consciousness) is associated to a neural state; it is impossible for there be a change of mental state without a corresponding change in neural state (Frith et al. 1999). Sometimes this assumption is referred to as the "supervenience thesis" of the mental on the physical (Kim 1998). Precise experimental settings and functional neuroimaging techniques allow us to place conscious properties within a biological framework (Delacour 1997; Edelman 2003). This led to the formulation of sophisticated theories about the neural correlates of visual consciousness and other conscious phenomena (Crick and Koch 1995; Kreiman et al. 2002). The neural correlates of consciousness can be defined as the minimal set of neuronal events that gives rise to a specific aspect of a conscious percept (Rees et al. 2002; Crick and Koch 2003). However, correlations between neural processes and features of conscious experience are far from providing a definitive explanation of the causal relationship between them (Fell et al. 2004). In spite of the remarkable progress and anticipated advances in the neurosciences in elucidating the neuronal mechanisms underlying mental states and cognitive functions, the identification of consciousness with these mechanisms avoids the subjective experience and fails to advance our understanding of consciousness (Dennett 2001). Therefore, the actual essence of the problem concerning consciousness is how any physical description can be synonymous with subjective experience. Or, in other words, how the subjective, first-person account of consciousness can be objectified in a somewhat reductive explanatory account (Churchland 1988; Chalmers 1998).

In this context, clinical neurosciences offer unique avenues for the understanding of the relationship between pathological brain function and altered conscious states. In this chapter the different ictal semiologies are demonstrated to illuminate certain neuroanatomical and neurophysiological facets of consciousness.

2.2. Level and Contents of Consciousness

Although a unified model encompassing all the wide spectrum of clinical alterations of consciousness seems hard to develop, a useful distinction can be made between the quantitative (level) and qualitative (content) features of consciousness (Frith et al. 1999; Plum and Posner 1980). We will introduce a bidimensional model for the description of physiological and pathological conscious states, which will provide a useful framework for the clinical pictures presented in the following chapters.

The level of consciousness is a matter of degree: a range of conscious and unconscious states extends from alert wakefulness through sleep into coma (Jones 1998; Young 1998). To be conscious in this sense means to be awake, aroused, or vigilant. The shift between the different levels of consciousness can easily be induced by exogenous substances, such as several drug classes acting on the central nervous system (Table 2.1). The level of consciousness can be quantified by analysing the behavioral responses that are constituent functions of consciousness as awareness. For example, the widely used Glasgow Coma Scale (GCS) adopted three objective parameters, namely motor responsiveness, speech, and eye opening, as measures to assess consciousness (see also chapter 4) (Teasdale and Jennett 1974). Interestingly enough, none of these faculties is either necessary or sufficient for consciousness (Crick et al. 2004).

Table 2.1. Main pathophysiological levels of consciousness and drug classes affecting them

Level of consciousness	Drug class
Excitement	Psychostimulants
Wakefulness	(normal state)
Drowsiness	Anxiolytics
Sleep	Hypnotics
Coma/vegetative states/anesthesia	Anesthetics

The ascending activating pontomesodiencephalic reticular formation, together with its thalamic targets, has been recognized as the principal substratum of vigilance since the pioneering works of Moruzzi and Magoun (1949). Circumscribed brain lesions involving the reticular formation and/or the thalamic intralaminar nuclei are associated with bilateral cortical impairment and therefore severe restrictions in the level of consciousness (Giacino 1997; Lee et al. 2002). Consequently, the upper brainstem-diencephalic activating system has been confirmed to represent the cornerstone of the neural substrates of conscious awareness (Ortinski and Meador 2004).

The second major dimension of consciousness is the content of subjective experience: sensations, emotions, memories, intentions and all the feelings that colour our inner world. This feature is determined by the interaction between exogenous factors derived from our environment and endogenous factors, such as attention (Coslett 1997). In the absence of diffuse cerebral dysfunction, the contents of consciousness reflect the specialized function performed by specific brain structures, in both physiological and pathological settings. Significant changes in consciousness contents have been elicited by early experiments of local electrical stimulation of human temporal cortex during epilepsy surgery (Jasper 1998; Penfield and Jasper 1954). In a similar way, the conscious recall of past events has been proven to require the integrity of medial temporal lobe structures (Penfield 1959; Gloor et al. 1982). During the last few years, neuroimaging studies have considerably deepened our understanding of the correlations between the contents of conscious states and the functional activation of selected cortical areas (Edelman 2003).

The relationship between level of arousal and contents of consciousness is complex and yet to be determined. The contents of consciousness can vary quite independently of the level of consciousness, as it has been demonstrated by specific cortical lesions altering the contents of consciousness without having any effects on the level of consciousness (Portas et al. 2004). On the other hand, the level of arousal has a major influence on the contents of consciousness. On the whole, as arousal increases, the extent and quality of conscious experience also increases; however, in peculiar pathological conditions, high levels of arousal can be associated with impoverished contents of consciousness (e.g. limbic status epilepticus – see chapter 5).

Figure 2.1 shows the bidimensional model of consciousness in a healthy subject, during the waking state. The level and contents of consciousness are plotted in a biaxial diagram, and dots indicate the possible conscious states of the subject according to these features. The level of consciousness during wakefulness is almost constantly elevated, while the contents of subjective experience show a greater variability.

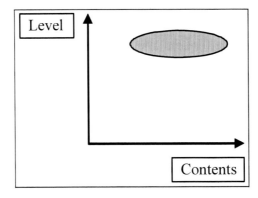

Figure 2.1. Bidimensional model of consciousness. Dots indicate conscious states in a healthy subject during wakefulness. Unlike the level of arousal, which is almost constantly high, the vividness of the contents of consciousness experienced in the wakeful state shows a wide degree of variability.

2.3. CONSCIOUSNESS WITHIN THE NEUROSCIENCES

2.3.1. John Eccles: Conscious Psychons

Australian neuropshysiologist John Eccles worked largely on the mechanisms of neurotransmission, for which he was awarded the Nobel prize for Physiology and Medicine in 1963. Over the course of several decades, partly in collaboration with the philosopher of science Sir Karl Popper, Eccles developed a theory of consciousness, known as interactionistic dualism. His basic philosophical starting point is the following:

"I maintain that the human mystery is incredibly demeaned by scientific reductionism, with its claim in promissory materialism to account eventually for all of the spiritual world in terms of patterns of neuronal activity. This belief must be classed as a superstition […] we have to recognize that we are spiritual beings with souls existing in a spiritual world as well as material beings with bodies and brains existing in a material world" (Eccles 1991).

Eccles' work on consciousness was largely motivated by the problem of the unity of experience: he came to the conclusion that "the unity of conscious experience is provided by the self-conscious mind and not by the neural machinery of the liaison areas of the cerebral hemisphere" (Popper and Eccles 1977). According to this view, the mind plays an active role in selecting, reading out and integrating neural activity, moulding it into a unified whole according to its desire or interest. The problem, as with all dualist theories, is to provide an explanation of how the separate mind carries out its selecting and unifying tasks, i.e. how this mind-brain interaction takes place.

Eccles embraced Popperian cosmology (Popper and Eccles 1977), which splits the universe into three interacting worlds: World 1 is the world of physical objects and events, including biological entities; World 2 is the world of mental objects and events (including consciousness); World 3 is the world of the products of the human mind, which contains abstract objects such as scientific theories, myths, art, social institutions, and so forth (Table 2.2).

Table 2.2. Popper and Eccles' ontology: description of the three worlds

World 1	World 2	World 3
Physical objects and states	Mental states	Knowledge
Inorganic matter	Memories	Cultural heritage coded on
Material artefacts	Dreams	material substrates
Energy of cosmos	Perceptions	Theoretical systems
Biological structures	Subjective experiences	incl. theories on
incl. brains	incl. consciousness	consciousness

Opponents of dualistic views argue that mind-brain interaction would infringe the law of the conservation of energy. Eccles (1994) showed that mind-brain action can be explained without violating the conservation of energy if account is taken of quantum physics and detailed knowledge of the microstructure of the neocortex. He called the fundamental neural units of the cerebral cortex "dendrons", and proposed that each of the 40 million dendrons is linked with a mental unit, or "psychon", representing a unitary conscious experience. In willed actions and thought, psychons act on dendrons and momentarily increase the probability of the firing of selected neurons, while in perception the reverse process takes place. Interaction among psychons themselves could explain the unity of our perceptions and of the inner world of our mind.

According to this theory, synapses in the cortex respond in a probabilistic manner to neural excitation, a probability that is governed by quantum uncertainty given the extremely small size of the synapsis' microsite that emits the neurotransmitter. Eccles speculated that an immaterial mind (in the form of psychons) controls the quantum "jumps" and turns them into voluntary excitations of the neurons that account for body motion (Eccles 1990; 1994).

Eccles felt that overall reductionistic/materialistic theories of consciousness failed to account for "the wonder and mystery of the human self with its spiritual values, with its creativity, and with its uniqueness for each of us" (Eccles 1994). He criticized these theories for allowing no real scope for human freedom. Though Eccles was motivated partly from his religious beliefs, it is clear from context that his concept of spirit was not confined to any particular religious or philosophical doctrine. That is, he equated the terms "spiritual" and "nonmaterial", which disengaged his thinking from Cartesian dualism and placed it in the path of modern science.

2.3.2. Francis Crick: The Astonishing Consciousness

The British biochemist and Nobel laureate Francis Crick made perhaps the clearest statement of a through-going reductionist approach to the problem of consciousness. In his own words, the "astonishing hypothesis" regarding consciousness reads as follows: "you, your joys and your sorrows, your memories and your ambitions, your sense of personal identity and free will, are in fact no more than the behaviour of a vast assembly of nerve cells and their associated molecules" (Crick 1994). Roughly speaking, Crick's statement means that conscious experience *is* the behaviour of neurons, rather than being caused by it, or interacting with it (Crick and Koch 1990; Koch 2006).

Crick studied consciousness mainly through the experimental paradigm of visual awareness and therefore was interested in consciousness that arises from external stimuli (Koch and Crick 1994). Awareness of something requires "attention" (being aware of one object rather than another), and attention requires "binding", since all the neurons that represent features of an object fire together to produce our conscious experience of the object. Crick believes that binding occurs through a synchronous (or correlated) firing of different regions of the brain. He subscribes to the view that synchronized firing in the range of 40 Hertz ("gamma oscillations") in the areas connecting the thalamus and the cortex might be the neural correlate of visual awareness.

Crick and Koch (1995; 2000) argued that, in the case of visual awareness, the neural correlate of consciousness must be an explicit, multi-level, symbolic interpretation of part of the visual scene. Explicitness implies that the neural correlate of consciousness must somehow refer to those features of the visual scene of which we are currently aware, for example, by a synchronized elevation of the firing rate of the cells which represent those features; moreover the neural correlate of consciousness for vision is likely to be multi-level in the sense that several levels of processing in the hierarchy of cortical visual areas are involved; finally, it is symbolic in the sense that there is a close correlation between features of the visual scene and the neural activity which represents them.

Crick's theory of visual awareness anticipates that the neural correlate of consciousness at any given time will involve a sparse but spatially distributed network of neurons, and that its activity must stand out above the background of neuronal firing for at least 100-200 ms. He suggested that the neuronal populations directly involved in the neural correlate of consciousness may have some unique combination of molecular, pharmacological, biophysical and anatomic properties: for example the "bursty" pyramidal cells in layer 5 of the cortical visual areas may play a critical role in the neural correlate of conscious vision. Moreover Crick proposed that neurons within area V1 (primary visual cortex), do not directly participate in the neural correlate of consciousness for visual awareness, despite supplying much of the information which is processed in visual areas downstream (Crick and Koch 1995). This idea has two sources: the empirical observation that several characteristics of our visual experience correlate more closely with the behavioural patterns of neurons in higher visual areas, such as area V4, than in V1; and the theoretical view that only cortical regions which can directly influence action, via interconnections with the frontal lobes, can contribute to consciousness.

Crick's theory has implications for the specific function of consciousness: it suggests that it may be more efficient for the brain to have one single explicit representation, instead of sending information, in tacit form, to many different parts of the brain. Crick explicitly stated that there is no separate "I" independent of neural firing (Crick and Koch 2003). His entire work can be seen as a magnificent attempt to get rid of our common-sense concept of the soul. With regards to subjectivity, he suggests that the best way to proceed in our seemingly endless way towards a theory of consciousness resides in the investigation of the neural correlates of consciousness (Crick 2004).

2.3.3. Gerald Edelman: The Darwinian Consciousness

According to Nobel Prize Gerald Edelman, consciousness is a natural development of the ability to build perceptual categories (e.g. "red", "pen", "cat"), the process that we normally call generalization. The brain can do this because neurons get organized by experience in maps, each neural map dealing with a feature of perceptions (color, shape, etc.). Edelman proposes a model which abstracts from the subjective properties of experience, from biological features of the thalamocortical networks which plausibly supply its contents, and from detailed computer simulations of their activity (Tononi and Edelman 1998). This model has a few key tenets (Edelman 2003). Basically, consciousness arises from the fast integration of a large amount of information within a "dynamic core" of strongly interacting elements. Re-entrying loops, via reciprocal interconnections between regions of the thalamocortical system, mediate this rapid integration. Built into the coalition theory is the theory of redundancy whereby the same representation (concept) can come about through the interaction of different populations of neurons (Edelman 1989; Edelman and Tononi 2000).

Edelman distinguishes between primary consciousness (imagery and sensations, i.e. being aware of things in the world) and higher-order consciousness (language and self-awareness). The emergence of primary consciousness and the construction of our multimodal perceptual world depend upon the integration of current sensory processing with previously acquired affect-laden memories. More specifically, primary consciousness requires (1) an active kind of memory, that does not simply store new information but also continuously reorganizes (or "recategorizes") old information; (2) the ability to learn, as a way to assign value to stimuli (a new value will result in a new behavior, and that is what learning is about); (3) the ability to make the distinction between the self and the rest of the world, i.e. a way to represent what is part of the organism and what is not. On the other hand, higher-order consciousness depends on re-entrant connections between language and conceptual systems. This allows for the construction of a coherent self-operating dynamic core, a large functional cluster that continuously changes, but maintains continuity and integration through its many reentrant loops. The dynamic core hypothesis avoids the need of any particular area, type of neuron, or firing rate, mysteriously to be conscious, while others are not. In addition, this model of a constantly shifting dynamic core of neural elements subserving consciousness accounts for many of its properties: its continuity and changefulness, its selectivity, the existence of a focus of attention and a more diffuse surround, its coherence, its pace of change and the wide access of its contents to other psychological operations (Edelman 1989; Edelman and Tononi 2000).

Edelman's theory plays down the role of particular neuronal types and cortical regions, but stresses the importance of the complex integration of thalamocortical subsystems which are both functionally segregated and highly interactive. Furthermore, rather than "space-based", this theory appears to be "process-based", since it is not only looking for the place where the self-referential feedback occurs, but also for the way it occurs, and the process turns out to be much more important than the place.

Central to Edelman's model is the theory of "neural Darwinism" or neuronal group selection (Edelman 1989; 2003; Edelman and Tononi 2000). Developmental selection occurs during the early development of the brain: neurons send out thousands of branches in all directions, providing enormous variability in connection patterns. Then, according to which connections are used and which not, certain connections are pruned in order to leave long-lasting functional groups. Thus, neuronal populations, which enlarge through competition, are matched to and supported by endogenous reward, memory, and self systems to form winning coalitions. Moreover, a similar process of "experiential selection" goes on throughout life: certain synapses within and between groups of locally coupled neurons are strengthened and others are weakened, without changes in macroscopic neuroanatomy. Edelman's theory of consciousness is based on selectionist principles, in that variant patterns are generated and selected, although there seems to be no mechanism for copying variants to make new ones.

Finally, from an evolutionary point of view, consciousness emerged when a category-value link emerged, that is when the basis for consciousness was laid (Edelman 2005). A higher-level consciousness (being aware of itself), probably unique to humans, is possible if the brain is also capable of abstracting the relationship between the self and the nonself through social interaction, and this leads naturally to the development of linguistic faculties. Edelman identifies the regions that are assigned to define self within a species (the amygdala, the hippocampus, the limbic system, the hypothalamus) and those that operate to define nonself (the cortex, the thalamus and the cerebellum). Notably, concept formation preceded language. With the advent of language, concepts became absolute, independent of time. In a similar fashion, semantics preceded syntax: acquiring phonological capacities provided the means for linking the preexisting conceptual operations with the emerging lexical operations. Thus, in Edelman's picture consciousness is exquisitely human, as only humans are able to think about the past and the future, whereas all animals are forced to live in the present, simply reacting to external and internal stimuli.

2.3.4. Antonio Damasio: Consciousness and Emotions

Portuguese neurologist Antonio Damasio distinguishes between two kinds of consciousness: core consciousness and extended consciousness. Core consciousness is the basic kind of consciousness and corresponds to the transient process that is incessantly generated relative to any object with which an organism interacts, and during which a transient core self and sense of knowing are automatically generated. Core consciousness is not exclusively human and requires neither language nor working memory, and needs only a brief short-term memory. Extended consciousness, on the other hand, is a more complex process. It depends on a set of self-referred conceptual memories pertaining to both past and anticipated experiences of the individual, and is enhanced by language faculties (Damasio 19994; 1999).

With regards to the problem of consciousness, Damasio splits it into two parts: the "movie in the brain" kind of experience (how a number of sensory inputs are transformed into the continuous flow of sensations of the mind) and the self (how the sense of "owning" that movie comes to be). Based on his studies of brain damaged patients, Damasio distinguishes between the proto-self, the core-self, and the autobiographical self. The proto-self is a set of neural patterns that map the state of an organism moment by moment. The core self is a transient entity, ceaselessy re-created for each and every object with which the brain interact. The autobiographical self depends on personal memories. Damasio is clear that this self is not any kind of separate entity but is the "you" that is born as the story of your life is told. The "I" is not telling the story: the "I" is created by stories told in the mind. As he puts in, "you are the music while the music lasts" (Damasio 1999).

For Damasio, consciousness is a "feeling", and feelings are neural patterns. His theory entails that neural patterns are displayed in the appropriate areas of the brainstem, thalamus, and cerebral cortex to generate the feelings. In turn, the display is not watched by other cerebral processes. Emotions also play a central role in Damasio's theory of consciousness. The Portuguese neurologist expands on the influence of somatic processes to the regulation of decision-making as well as emotion in his influential somatic marker hypothesis (Damasio 1994; Dunn et al. 2006). The somatic marker hypothesis proposes that "somatic marker" biasing signals from the body are represented and regulated in the emotion circuitry of the brain, particularly the ventromedial prefrontal cortex, to help regulate decision-making in situations of complexity and uncertainty (e.g Damasio 1996). In his *Looking for Spinoza* (2003) Damasio uses the philosopher Baruch Spinoza as his foil for developing a detailed theory of human feelings and emotions in both neurobiological and neuroanatomic terms.

The core concept of *Looking for Spinoza* is the difference between emotions and feelings both as individual cognitive processes and as model systems for consciousness in general. In Damasio's account, emotion is the physical response to certain environmental stimuli and is a universal response available to many organisms. Feelings are the conscious correlate of the emotional reaction and are present in few species. In this system, feelings are part of the hard problem of consciousness. According to Damasio, feelings and emotions (such as anger) are part of the body's way of recognizing deviations away from homeostatic set-points toward which the body would eventually like to return, and which result in a set of reactions that cause this to happen.

In Damasio's model, bodily representations, the substrate for feelings and emotions, are mediated by a series of well-detailed brain structures including the insular cortex, and are necessary for conscious perception. These "self" structures are modified by the internal representations of external sensory stimuli and, through recursive brain neuroanatomy, this interaction becomes available as conscious perception. Finally, Damasio points out that emotional underpinnings led to the development of group interaction through compromise.

Education, in particular, and society, in general, are described as important means to modulate emotional responses and maintain societal constructs.

2.3.5. Bernard Baars: A Workspace for Consciousness

Psycholinguist Bernard Baars developed a rigorous theoretical model of consciousness that borrowed from and expanded on the notion of parallel distributed processing. According to this model, the nervous system is viewed as a distributed collection of specialized parallel processors, which cooperate and compete for the access to an integrative domain called a "global workspace" (Baars 1988; 2005). These specialized processors, which are thought to be largely unconscious, broadcast messages to the other processors just as if they were writing on a blackboard visible to every other agent. On the other hand, the blackboard functions represent the global workspace of consciousness. Any conscious experience emerges from cooperation and competition between the many processing units of the brain working in parallel. In other words, Baars' model identifies the contents of consciousness with the contents of the global workspace, which can be broadcast widely through the nervous system, to recruit the operation of the numerous unconscious specialized subsystems to the task in hand.

Baars emphasizes that conscious and unconscious processes are vastly different: unconscious processes are highly efficient in their own specialized tasks (characterized by low errors, high speed, almost unlimited capacity, and little mutual interference); conscious processes are computationally inefficient (characterized by high errors, low speed, very limited capacity, and mutual interference). Whereas unconscious processes are relatively isolated, autonomous in reference to each other, and have limited range over time, conscious processes can relate conscious contents to each other rather easily, and hence have a great range of different contents over time (Baars 1988).

For Baars, the definition of a processor is recursive. A processor is usually part of a structured coalition of processors, and can be functionally decomposable into many components. Therefore, functionally separable processors can only be defined momentarily, within the context of a single task – in some other task or context, processors may be rearranged in some other way; perhaps in a different organization they are functionally inseparable from a superordinate processor (Baars 1987). This means that different processors may be superprocessors or subprocessors, depending on the task at hand and the cerebral circuitry involved. Although such a definition complicates theoretical matters making the definition of processors somewhat circular, it does give high flexibility to the system, a flexibility akin to that of the human consciousness (Baars 1997).

The global workspace theory emphasizes a two-way flow between conscious and unconscious brain activities. The theory has been implemented in large-scale computational and neural net models and bears a close resemblance to Edelman's model of neural Darwinism. Baars suggests that it is helpful to think metaphorically of a theater of mind (Baars 1997; 2002). In the conscious spotlight on stage – the global workspace – an actor speaks, and his words and gestures are distributed to many unconscious audience members, sitting in the darkened hall. Different listeners understand the performance in different ways.

But as the audience claps or boos in response, the actor can change his words, or walk off to yield to the next performer. Finally, behind the scenes, an invisible (unconscious) director and playwright try to exercise executive control over the actor and the spotlight.

Less metaphorically, information appears to flow into a neuronal global workspace to be widely distributed. Such a structure must combine converging inputs – the actors competing for access to the spotlight – followed by momentary dominance of one coherent input, and then wide distribution of output, in a wave of activity sent to other regions. In the brain, the reticular-thalamic system behaves like a global workspace in a parallel distributed system. The reticular-thalamic system incorporates the classical brainstem reticular formation, the non-specific nuclei of the thalamus, and the fibers that project, in diffuse fashion, upward from the thalamus to "activate" the cortex. The reticular-thalamic system, along with the interlinked frontoparietal association cortices, are involved in wakefulness, the orienting response, the focus of attention, and the most central integrative processes of the brain. In Baars' words, "there is considerable neurophysiological evidence to suggest that the reticular-thalamic system is the major substrate of conscious experience, while the cortex and perhaps other parts of the brain may provide the content of conscious experience" (Baars 1987).

2.4. THE NEUROPSYCHIATRY OF CONSCIOUSNESS

Ancient Greek philosopher disputed whether the seat of consciousness was in the lungs, in the heart, or in the brain. The brain's pre-eminence is now undisputed, and scientists are trying to establish which specific parts of the brain belong to the neural network correlates of conscious experiences. In fact, the basic premise that all human sensation, emotion, motivation, volition are products of brain function, underlies contemporary approaches to understanding human behavior and the effects of brain dysfunction in the clinical discipline of neuropsychiatry. This brain-based approach acknowledges that the environmental influences (interpersonal relationships, social and cultural influences, etc.) are mediated through central nervous system structures and function. For every deviant environmental event there will be a corresponding change in central nervous system function, and when central nervous system function is altered there will be corresponding changes in the behavior or subjective experience of the individual (Cummings 1996). Neuropsychiatry is the clinical discipline devoted to understanding the neurobiological basis, optimal assessment, natural history, and most efficacious treatment of disorders of the nervous system with such manifestations (Cummings and Hegarty 1994).

The last few decades have seen an incredible advance in neuroscience applicable to neuropsychiatry. Studies in genetics and molecular biology have revealed mutations that cause major neuropsychiatric disturbances. Moreover, advances in structural and functional imaging techniques have been particularly important in the growth of neuropsychiatry, by providing critical information about brain function in neuropsychiatric illnesses associated with impairment of consciousness. Together, these technologies provide a diverse armamentarium of techniques for diagnosing central nervous system disease and understanding their pathophysiology. Progress in neuropsychology also informs contemporary neuropsychiatry. There have been substantial advances, for example, in recognizing and characterizing how focal brain lesions and diffuse degenerative disorders differentially affect cognitive processes, depending on the brain structures involved. Several conditions are now much better understood as a result of the application of basic science. Idiopathic neuropsychiatric illnesses have been the subject of intensive scientific scrutiny over the last few years: regional changes in brain structure have been identified and genetic and environmental contributors to the syndromes discovered. From a clinical perspective, this improved understanding of basic disease processes facilitates identification and interpretation of the clinical syndromes and provides a basis for the development of therapeutic agents. The success of biological treatment of neuropsychiatric disorders implies that neurotransmitter disturbances are involved in the mediation of behavioral and consciousness disturbances (Trimble 1996).

By definition, neuropsychiatry includes both the psychiatric manifestations of neurologic illness and neurobiology of idiopathic psychiatric disorders (Cummings and Hegarty 1994). Brain disorders, unlike their medical counterparts, are manifest by alterations in behaviors and subjective experiences: in many ways they are disorders of the person rather than disorders that happen to the individual. Neuropsychiatry provides principles of brain-behavior relationships and a means of understanding human private experience. Study of brain-behavior relationships and neuropsychiatric syndromes provides insight into abstract concepts such as self and culture, allows understanding of the neurobiological basis of human behavior both individually and in the context of an evolving culture, and allows construction of a neuroepistemology (Cummings 1996). Finally, based on these assumptions, neuropsychiatry offers a privileged clinical perspective on the putative neural bases of normal and altered conscious states (Hamanaka 1997). This volume presents a contemporary view of the neuropsychiatric approach to the problem of consciousness and the advances in clinical and basic neuroscience applicable to understanding and interpreting human conscious experience.

2.5. REFERENCES

Baars BJ. *A cognitive theory of consciousness.* Cambridge, UK: Cambridge University Press 1988.

Baars BJ. *In the theatre of consciousness.* New York: Oxford University Press 1997.

Baars BJ. Global workspace theory of consciousness: evidence, theory, and some phylogenetic speculations. In: Greenberg G, Tobach E, eds. *Cognition, language, and consciousness: integrative levels.* Hillsdale, New Jersey: Lawrence Erlbaum 1987.

Baars BJ. Global workspace theory of consciousness: toward a cognitive neuroscience of human experience. *Prog Brain Res.* 2005;150:45-53.

Baars BJ. The conscious access hypothesis: origins and recent evidence. *Trends Cogn Sci.* 2002;6: 47-52.

Chalmers D. The problems of consciousness. *Adv Neurol* 1998;77:7-18.

Churchland PS. Reduction and the neurobiological basis of consciousness. In: Marcel AJ, Bisiach E, editors. *Consciousness in contemporary science*. Oxford: Oxford University Press; 1988. p. 273-304.

Coslett HB. Consciousness and attention. *Semin Neurol* 1997;17:137-144.

Crick FC, Koch C, Kreiman G, Fried I. Consciousness and neurosurgery. *Neurosurgery* 2004;55:273-282.

Crick FC, Koch C. A framework for consciousness. *Nature Neurosci* 2003;6:119-126.

Crick FC, Koch C. Are we aware of neural activity in primary visual cortex? *Nature* 1995;375:121-123.

Crick FC, Koch C. Consciousness and neuroscience. *Cereb Cortex* 1998;8:97-107.

Crick FC, Koch C. *The unconscious homunculus.* In: Metzinger T, ed. *The neural correlates of consciousness.* Cambridge, MA: MIT Press 2000.

Crick FC, Koch C. Towards a neurobiological theory of consciousness. *Semin Neurosci* 1990;2:263-276.

Crick FC, Koch C. What are the neural correlates of consciousness? In: Van Hemmen L, Sejnowski TJ, editors. *Problems in systems neuroscience.* New York: Oxford University Press; 2003. p. 273-282.

Crick FC. *The astonishing hypothesis: the scientific search for the soul.* New York: Simon and Schuster 1994.

Cummings JL, Hegarty A. Neurology, psychiatry, and neuropsychiatry. *Neurology.* 1994;44:209-213.

Cummings JL. Neuropsychiatry and society. *J Neuropsychiatry Sci.* 1996;8:104-109.

Damasio A. *Descartes' error: emotion, reason, and the human brain.* New York: GP Putnam 1994.

Damasio A. *The feeling of what happens: body and emotion in the making of consciousness.* New York, NY: Hartcourt Brace 1999.

Damasio A. *Looking for Spinoza: joy, sorrow, and the feeling brain.* New York, NY: Hartcourt Brace 2003.

Dunn BD, Dalgleish T, Lawrence AD. The somatic marker hypothesis: a critical evaluation. *Neurosci Biobehav Rev.* 2006;30:239-271.

Delacour J. Neurobiology of consciousness: an overview. *Behav Brain Res* 1997;85:127-141.

Dennett D. Are we explaining consciousness yet? *Cognition* 2001;79:221-237.

Eccles JC. A unitary hypothesis of mind-brain interaction in the cerebral cortex, *Proc Roy Soc London B.* 1990;240:433-51.

Eccles JC. *Evolution of the Brain, Creation of the Self.* New York: Routledge 1991.

Eccles JC. *How the Self Controls its Brain.* Berlin: Springer-Verlag 1994.

Edelman GM. Naturalizing consciousness: a theoretical framework. *Proc Natl Acad Sci USA.* 2003;100:5520-24.

Edelman GM. *The remembered present: a biological theory of consciousness.* New York: Basic Books 1989.

Edelman GM. *Wider than the sky: the phenomenal gift of consciousness.* Yale: Yale University Press 2005.

Edelman GM, Tononi G. *A universe of consciousness.* New York: Basic Books 2000.

Fell J, Elger CE, Kurthen M. Do neural correlates of consciousness cause conscious states? *Med Hypotheses* 2004;63:367-369.

Flanagan O. Consciousness and the natural method. *Neuropsychologia* 1995;33:1103-1115.

Frith C, Perry R, Lumer E. The neural correlates of conscious experience: an experimental framework. *Trends Cogn Sci* 1999;3:105-114.

Giacino JT. Disorders of consciousness: differential diagnosis and neuropathological features. *Semin Neurol* 1997;17:105-111.

Gloor P, Olivier A, Quesney LF, Andermann F, Horowitz S. The role of the limbic system in experiential phenomena of temporal lobe epilepsy. *Ann Neurol* 1982;12:129-144.

Hamanaka T. The concept of consciousness in the history of neuropsychiatry. Hist Psychiatry 1997;8:361-373.

Jasper HH. Sensory information and conscious experience. *Adv Neurol* 1998;77:33-48.

Jones BE. The neural basis of consciousness across the sleep-waking cycle. *Adv Neurol* 1998;77:75-94.

Kim J. *Mind in a physical world*. Cambridge, MA: MIT Press; 1998.

Koch C, Crick F. Some further ideas regarding the neuronal basis of awareness. In Koch C, Davis JL, eds. *Large-scale neuronal theories of the brain*. Cambridge: MIT Press 1994.

Koch C. *The quest for consciousness: a neurobiological approach*. Englewood: Roberts & Co. 2004.

Kreiman G, Fried I, Koch C. Single-neuron correlates of subjective vision in the human medial temporal lobe. *Proc Natl Acad Sci USA* 2002;99:8378-8383.

Lee KH, Meador KJ, Park YD, King DW, Murro AM, Pillai JJ, Kaminski RJ. Pathophysiology of altered consciousness during seizures: subtraction SPECT study. *Neurology* 2002;59:841-846.

Moruzzi G, Magoun HW. Brain stem reticular formation and the activation of the EEG. *Electroencephalogr Clin Neurophysiol* 1949;455-473.

Ortinski P, Meador KJ. Neuronal mechanisms of conscious awareness. *Archives of Neurology* 2004;61:1017-1020.

Penfield W, Jasper H. *Epilepsy and the functional anatomy of the human brain*. Boston: Little, Brown; 1954.

Penfield W. The interpretive cortex: the stream of consciousness in the human brain can be electrically reactivated. *Science* 1959;129:1719-1725.

Plum F, Posner JB. *The diagnosis of stupor and coma*. Philadelphia: Davis; 1980.

Popper K, Eccles J. *The self and its brain*. New York: Springer 1977.

Portas C, Maquet P, Rees G, Blakemore S, Frith C. The neural correlates of consciousness. In: Frackowiak RSJ, Friston KJ, Frith CD, Dolan RJ, Price CJ, Zeki S, Ashburner J, Penny W, editors. *Human brain function*. San Diego, CA: Academic Press; 2004.

Rees G, Kreiman G, Koch C. Neural correlates of consciousness in humans. *Nat Rev Neurosci* 2002;3:261-270.

Searle J. Consciousness. *Annu Rev Neurosci* 2000;23:557-578.

Searle J. How to study consciousness scientifically. *Philos Trans R Soc Lond B* 1998;353:1935-42.

Teasdale G, Jennett B. Assessment of coma and impaired consciousness: a practical scale. *Lancet* 1974;2:81-84.

Tononi G, Edelman G. Consciousness and complexity. *Science.* 1998;282:1846-51.

Trimble MR. *Biological psychiatry.* Chichester: John Wiley & Sons 1996.

Young GB. *Coma and impaired consciousness: a clinical perspective.* New York: McGraw-Hill; 1998.

Zeman A. *Consciousness: a user's guide.* London: Yale University Press; 2003.

Chapter 3

WAKEFULNESS AND SLEEP

At pater e populo natorum mille quorum
Excitat artificem simulatoremque figurae
Morphea.

(From the crowds of the thousands of his sons
Sleep called to himself Morpheus, master
In representing figures)

Ovid, Metamorphosis XI, vv. 635-636

3.1. THE MYSTERIES OF SLEEP

No other physiological phenomenon of human life is more intriguing and fascinating than sleep, and the literary and artistic quotations about sleep and its mysterious relationship with death are as old as the world. In the Talmud (Berakot 576) it is written: "Sleep is the sixtieth part (i.e. a fragment) of death" Doubtlessly, sleeping is the only physiological experience, in the living being, during which consciousness is lost, but it will soon be resumed, and this happens in a continuous cyclic fashion for the whole life. Another relevant feature of sleep is that it allows us to rest and recover from the fatigue of each day, as if entering into the dark tunnel of the loss of consciousness would *per se* represent a time to eliminate the excess of sensorial inputs accumulated during the daily conscious existence. It stands therefore necessary and mandatory to investigate scientifically sleep under all aspects (neurophysiological, neuroradiological, neurochemical and so on), in order to understand what happens in the brain when consciousness is lost and so, indirectly, speculate about the basic mechanisms underlying brain function during wakefulness, i.e. when full consciousness is present.

In a very simplistic way, sleep is recognizable by its contrast to wakefulness, and its second feature is motor inhibition. The third characteristic which differentiates sleep from most states of altered consciousness is that it is promptly reversibile. However, the border between sleep and wakefulness is not sharp, as the transition between the two phases often lasts several minutes and the precise moment of falling asleep may be impossibile to determine. Similarly, awakening may be sudden or gradual. Consciousness itself is a graded characteristic of mental activity. Conscious states fluctuate continuously between waking and dreaming: between these extremes there is a continuum of states which explains phenomena such as hypnosis, fantasy, concentration, etc. It has been claimed that the three fundamental states of consciousness are waking, sleeping and dreaming (Hobson et al. 2000). This chapter encompasses the different neurobiological aspects of these states and their relationship with conscious experiences.

3.2. REGULATION OF THE SLEEP-WAKE CYCLE

The second half of 19th century has seen an enormous growth of studies on sleep and sleep disorders, so that it seemed necessary to create a new superspecialized branch of medicine ad hoc defined "*sleep medicine*" (Chokroverty 1999; Shneerson 2005). The most relevant acquisitions on the physiology of sleep have been achieved over the last 50 years by means of polisomnography, i.e. the simultaneous recordings during sleep of the electroencephalographic tracing (EEG), muscle tone and activity (EMG), ocular movements (oculography), body movements (actigraphy), heart and lung rhythms, and a number of other physiological variables, such as blood pressure and oxyhaemoglobine saturation.

3.2.1. Sleep Architecture

The first fundamental distinction that has to be done is that there are two sleep patterns: non-REM and REM (rapid eye movements) sleep (Figure 3.1 and Table 3.1). Non-REM sleep is divided into four stages, which, from the first to the fourth one, show a progressive slowing of brain electrical activity (from 5.7 to 0.5-3 Hz). In particular, stage 1 is characterized by a fragmentation and a slowing down of normal alpha rhythm, with the appearance at EEG of the so called "*vertex sharp waves*" and transients, represented by both spikes (less than 70 ms duration) and sharp waves (more than 70 ms duration).

Table 3.1. Normal phases of human sleep

non-REM sleep	Orthodox sleep
	Synchronized sleep
	Quiet sleep (in infants)
non-REM sleep (stages 1 and 2)	Light sleep
non-REM sleep (stages 3 and 4)	Delta sleep
	Slow-wave sleep
REM sleep	Paradoxical sleep
	Desynchronized sleep
	Active sleep (in infants)

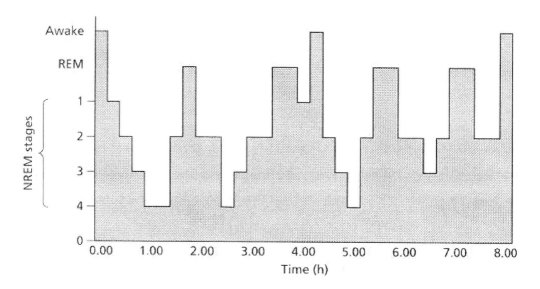

Figure 3.1. Sleep architecture: normal adult hypnogram.

In stage 2 particular biphasic events (*K complexes*) appear, along with the so called "sleep spindles", while stages 3 and 4 are characterized by theta and delta EEG rhythms, and are called "*slow sleep*" and "*deep sleep*" stages, due to the greater difficulties encountered in waking up (Figures 3.2 to 3.7).

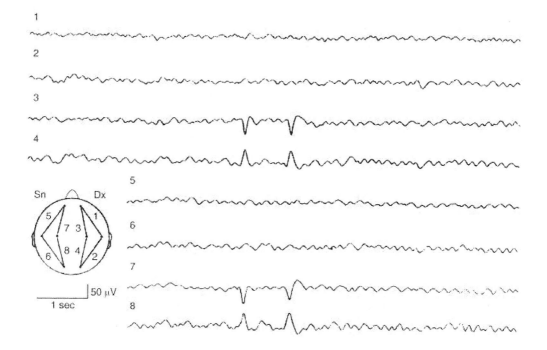

Figure 3.2. EEG pattern: non-REM sleep, stage 1.

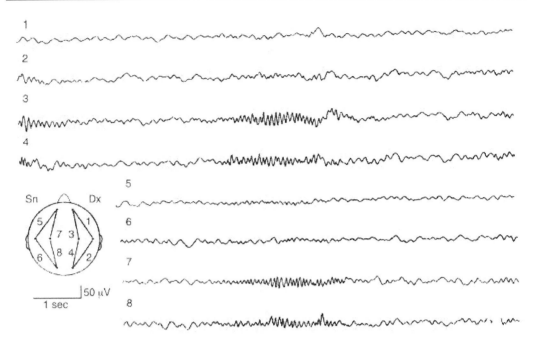

Figure 3.3. EEG pattern: non-REM sleep, stage 2.

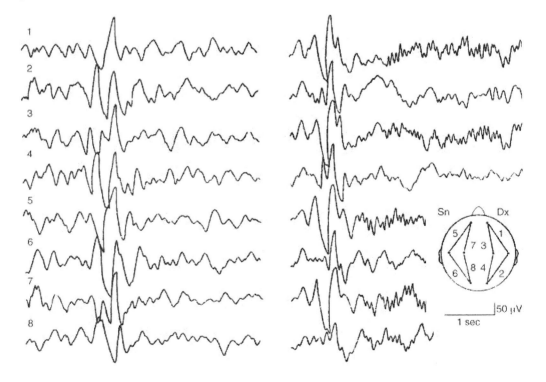

Figure 3.4. EEG pattern: non-REM sleep, stage 2 (K complexes).

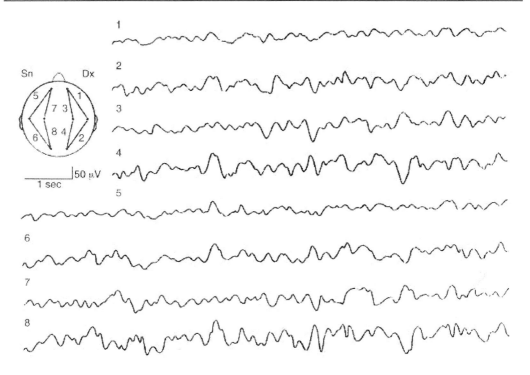

Figure 3.5. EEG pattern: non-REM sleep, stage 3.

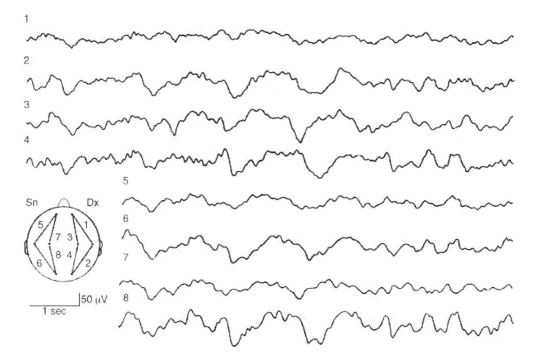

Figure 3.6. EEG pattern: non-REM sleep, stage 4.

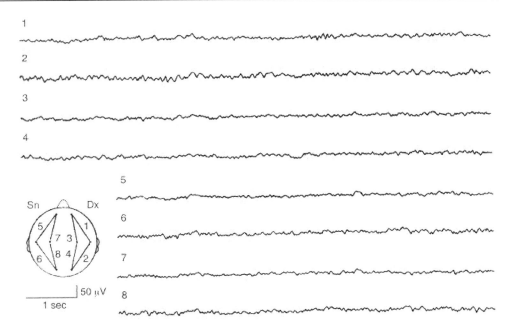

Figure 3.7. EEG pattern: REM sleep.

During the non-REM sleep there is a decrease of muscular tone, eyes are fixed, blood pressure and heart rate decrease. REM sleep, on the other hand, is characterized by low voltage brain electrical activiy, quite similarly to open eye wakefulness. Depth EEG recordings show discontinuous action potentials in the dorsal pons, lateral geniculate nucleus and occipital cortex (*ponto-geniculo-occipital spikes, PGO*). PGO spikes are normally synchronous with rapid eye movements and are important in determining basic sleep mechanisms. Muscular tone further decreases, with the exception of respiratory and ocular muscles, and eyes show low movements interrupted by bursts of rapid movements in every direction. Blood pressure and heart rate increase, and in man penile erections develop rapidly, and may persist during non-REM sleep. The termoregulatory system is grossly impaired. Within the REM sleep are concentrated most of those peculiar psychic activities/experiences that we call "dreams", especially the visual ones.

Dreams are present also in non-REM sleep, although in a more variable pattern and shorter duration. About 10-70% of subjects woken up during non-REM sleep will refer that they were actually dreaming, and the percentage goes up to 80% of subjcts in case of REM sleep, also including the ones who affirm that they do not usually dream. Non-REM and REM sleep alternate during the night. In falling asleep (drowsiness), there is a non-REM phase, which develops through stages 1-4, which may be followed by after 70-110 minutes by a REM phase. Cycles may be 4-5 per night. As sleep deepens, stages 3 and 4 of non-REM sleep become shorter, while REM sleep stages get longer. The organization of cycles and the proportion of phases vary according to the age of the subject, and such variation is better appreciated in the extreme ages of life - see, for instance, the need of a daytime nap. Another important phenomenon is the shortening of total sleep duration in the elderly (for an extensive review on all of the above see also Kryger et al. 2000; Shneerson 2005).

The staging criteria for sleep, originally outlined by Rechtschaffen and Kales in 1969, have been recently updated by the American Academy of Sleep Medicine (AASM). According to the 2007 AASM standards, non-REM sleep consists of stages N1 to N4. During Stage N1 the brain transitions from alpha to theta waves. This stage is sometimes referred to as somnolence, or drowsy sleep. Associated with the onset of sleep during N1 may be sudden twitches and hypnic jerks. During N1 the subject loses some muscle tone and conscious awareness of the external environment. Stage N2 is characterized by EEG patterns of sleep spindles and K-complexes, and occupies 45–55% of total sleep time. During this stage conscious awareness of the external environment completely disappears. Stages N3 and N4 are the deepest forms of sleep; N4 is effectively a deeper version of N3, in which the deep-sleep characteristic, such as delta-waves, are more pronounced. REM sleep (Stage R, or Stage 5) is associated with dreaming and can occur during all other stages of sleep. REM sleep is predominant in the final third of a sleep period; the EEG in this stage is aroused and looks similar to stage 1, and sometimes includes beta waves.

3.2.2. Neuroanatomical and Neurophysiological Bases of Sleep

The understanding of the basic mechanisms of sleep began with the pioneering experiments of Moruzzi and Magoun (1949) in the Laboratory of Pisa, who showed that the electrical stimulation of the brainstem reticular formation in the cat was able to provoke an "arousal" reaction, whereas the destruction of this area was associated with a comatous state followed by a long-term reduction of total wakefulness hours. These neuronal areas were therefore able to play a promoting or sustaining role of the wakefulness state. According to their theory, sleep was conceived as a passive phenomen. Ten years later, the first "coup de theatre" occurred, as the same working group was able to show that the midbrain reticular formation was under the physiological inhibitory influence of another portion of the same reticular formation, located in the bulbopontine area. In fact, disconnecting the two areas by means of a lesion at the pons level (pretrigeminal mediopontine and pretrigeminal hemipontine preparations: Batini et al. 1959; Cordeau and Mancia 1959), they obtained an animal which was in a continuous state of awakefulness, thus establishing that the brainstem reticular formation was a complex structure with both hypnogenic and awakening functions. Sleep was therefore no longer considered a passive phenomemon, but an active one.

Further studies were then able to demonstrate that also the stimulation of posterior hypothalamus, just rostral to midbrain reticular formation, causes arousal (Sherin et al. 1996). In this case, the neurons involved are of the histaminergic type and have axons that are directd either rostrally toward the midbrain or caudally to forebrain. This system explains the well known hypnotic effect of most antihistaminic drugs. On the other hand, the electrical stimulation of anterior hypothalamus and nearby areas of basal forebrain rapidly induces sleep, whereas their lesion causes a reduction of long lasting sleep (Saper et al. 2001). It is believed that the hypnotic action of this brain structure is mediated by GABAergic inhibitory neurons, named "*non-REM-on cells*"(Nitz and Siegel 1997a and b). These particular cells would cause sleep by inhibition of the histaminergic system above described and the cells of the reticular nucleus of oral pons, i.e. of those structures at the border between pons and midbrain that mediate wakefulness and sleep.The non-REM-on system is especially active, as expected, during the non-REM sleep, while it turns to be inactive during wakefulness and REM sleep. Most of these cells are activated by heat, and this might explain the known sleep-promoting effect of moderately elevated temperature.

Spindles and slow waves that characterize the EEG pattern of REM sleep are produced by synchronized postsynaptic potentials in neurons of diffuse cortical areas. This process of synchronization depends on the rhythmic discharge of GABA-ergic neurons that form the so-called thalamic reticular nucleus, which "*grosso modo*" surrounds the thalamus in a shell-like fashion.These neurons show a particular kind of discharge, which represents a crucial event in the generation of EEG spindles, and which is characterized by the cyclic alternation of membrane hyperpolarization and action potential bursts secondary to massive calcium ion influx into neurons. Actually, it is the hyperpolarization itself to determine the calcium influx, which causes the opening of related voltage-dependent channels. At the end of the calcium-mediated burst, membrane currents behave in such a way to go back to the hyperpolarization state, so that the cycle resumes (Huguenard 1998). The reticular nuclus projects to thalamocortical neurons, thus forcing them to a similar regimen of rhythmic discharges, which at once is translated into cortical postsynaptic potentials. These latter appear at the EEG as "*sleep spindles*". The massive involvement of this activity of thalamocortical neurons precludes, at the same time, that they may vehiculate, as in wakefulness, sensory inputs to cortex, which therefore remains "isolated" from the environment.

On the other hand, during REM sleep the EEG spindle and low wave activity disappears completely, and in this case an important role is played by the structures of the reticular substance of dorsal pons and midbrain, where there are abundant cholinergic cells. These are wakefulness-promoting areas, which have been shown to be active also in REM sleep (Vazquez and Baghdoyan 2000). Their axons actually project to the neurons of the thalamic reticular nucleus, depolarizing them and thus inhibiting the opposite process of hyperpolarization, which is the basic event of rhythmic thalamocortical activity. The last one is then replaced by an asynchronous activity, which eventually results in the typical low-voltage EEG patterns of this phase. Within the pontomesencephalic reticular formation, the physiological role of the reticular nucleus of oral pons is well recognised, as its bilateral destructionis known to abolish REM sleep for long periods. The neurons of this area are sensitive to acetylcholine and receive relevant cholinergic projections from nearby (dorsal and lateral) regions of reticular formation. They are at least three groups of neurons within this nucleus. The so-called *PGO (pontogeniculo-occipital)-on cells* are cholinergic neurons that project to the lateral geniculate nucleus, thus originating the PGO spike activity which are typical of REM sleep. The PGO-on cells are in turn regulated by the so-called *REM-off-cells*, coming from the median raphe nuclei and using serotonin as neurotransmitter (Bentivoglio and Steriade 1990). During wakefulness, these cells hyperpolarize and therefore prevent the burst discharge of PGO-on cells. They are important even when inactive. Other brainstem cellular groups show similar activity to REM-off cells, in particular noradrenergic neurons of the locus coeruleus and histaminergic neurons of posterior hypothalamus. It is likely that the interruption of the activity of these cellular regions represents a crucial event in many physiological changes that are typical of REM sleep. In the reticular nucleus of oral pons there are also *REM-waking-on cells*, that are active during both wakefulness and REM sleep. Some of them project toward the alpha spinal motor neurons, while others send projections to oculomotor nuclei, and it seems that the last ones are responsible for the rapid eye movements phenomenon, after which the REM phase is named (Reinoso Suarez et al. 2001). A third class of nuclear cells are the so-called *REM-on cells*, that are highly active exclusively during REM sleep, while they are inactive in wakefulness or during non-REM sleep. A subtype of these cells is certainly of the GABAergic kind and is responsible for inhibition of serotonergic and noradrenergic activities observed during REM sleep. A further glutamatergic subtype is responsible for the loss of muscular tone. Such loss is due to an active inhibitory process of alpha motor neurons belonging to motor nuclei, by the interposition of descending glycinergic system proceeding from pontine and bulbar structures. The function of REM-on cells has been investigated by experiments of microlesions of the reticular nucleus of the oral pons, in order to release, in the animal, the motor activity normally suppressed during REM sleep. In this case, the animal might accompany the dreams with movements. A human correlate of this condition might be represented by REM sleep behavioral disturbances, in which dreams "are vividly lived" (see Pace-Schott and Hobson 2002 for extensive review).

3.2.3. Circadian Rhythms

The circadian rhythms (24 hours) are generated by an internal pacemaker, oscillator or biological clock, whose activity is modified by external factors (time givers, cues or "*zeitgebers*"). These either reset or entrain the internal clock and gear it to the external environment. The suprachiasmatic nucleus (SCN) in the supra-optic region of the anterior hypothalamus is the centre responsible for the most important circadian rhythms, which in humans range between 23.5 and 24.5 hours. The SCN has a core of neurons which secrete either vaso-intestinal peptide or gastro-releasing peptide. They respond particularly to light stimuli via the retino-hypothalamic tract and have melatonin receptors. The "shell" of arginine-vasopressin and calretinin-releasing neurons respond to non-photic stimuli. The cells of the SCN are capable of spontaneous depolarization. The coordination of these is the source of circadian rhythmicity, but within the SCN there are subpopulations of cells with different cycle times (Russell and Gelder 2004). The SCN is active during the day, and in humans promotes wakefulness and influences the structures which control the onset and maintenance of sleep, but is not solely responsible for this. Impulses reach the SCN from retinal receptors (retinal ganglion cells), travelling in the retino-hypothalamic tract, which runs within the optic nerve to monosynaptically reach the SCN. Other impules from the retinal ganglion cells reach the pretectum, superior colliculus and sub-paraventricular zone. These probably mediate the pupillary light reflex and the effects of light exposure on non-REM and REM sleep, but do not lead any visual sensation (Espana and Scammell 2004). The cholinergic peducolopontine and laterodorsal tegmental (LDT/PPT) nuclei and basal forebrain neurons also project to the SCN, as do the ascending reticular activating system and other areas of the brainstem. Fibres leave the SNC to reach the ventrolateral preoptic area (VLPO) of the anterior hypothalamus multisynaptically. Other fibres also travel from the SCN to the hypothalamus, to control pituitary function, to the thalamus, the medial preoptic nucleus and multisynaptically to the pineal gland, whose most important hormone is melatonin (Brzezinski 1997).

3.3. Neurotransmitters of Sleep

Overall, aminergic and cholinergic neurons of the mesopontine junction interact in a way that results in the ultradian (less than 24 hours) alternation of mammalian REM and non-REM sleep (Hobson et al. 1975). In this model, REM-on cells of the pontine reticular formation are cholinergically excitatory at their synaptic endings. Pontine REM-off cells are noradrenergically or serotoninergically inhibitory. During waking, the pontine aminergic system is tonically activated and inhibits the pontine cholinergic system. During non-REM sleep, aminergic inhibition decreases progressively and cholinergic inhibition increases. At REM sleep onset, aminergic inhibition is shut off, and cholinergic excitability peaks while every other output is inhibited. Intermediate synaptic steps might however intervene in the initiation and augmentation of REM at the level of both REM-on mesopontine neurons and REM-off pontine aminergic nuclei (Leonard 1994).

Other neurotransmitters modulate the REM/non-REM system (Saper 2001). Dopamine has complex effects on wakefulness and sleep. Dopaminergic neurons from the substantia nigra radiate to the striatum, nucleus accumbens and, indirectly, to the prefrontal cortex. They increase alertness, modify motor activity and have sympathetic-like effects. Mesolimbic tract neurons project to the prefrontal and limbic cortex, particularly the amygdala and hippocampus, and are associated with arousal, and cognitive and emotional functions.

Histamine promotes wakefulness and arousal, and it is a transmitter of a system originating in neurons of the tuberomammillary nucleus (TMN) of the posterior hypothalamus, which projects widely to the ventrolateral preoptic area (VLPO), locus coeruleus, raphe nuclei, and laterodorsal tegmental (LDT) and peducolopontine tegmental (PPT) nuclei. The mutual inhibition of the VLPO and TMN is thought to be responsible for the osciillation between sleep and wakefulness (Saper 2001).

Gamma-aminobutyric acid (GABA) and glutamate also influence the REM/non-REMcycle. GABA-A receptors are primarily involved in promoting sleep, and GABAergic neurons are widespread in the brainstem reticular formation, hypothalamus and thalamus. GABA release from the VLPO inhibits the aminergic wakefulness-promoting nuclei (Nitz and Siegel 1997a and b).

Glutamate interacts with cholinergic and cholinoceptive neurons to generate the exponential increase in mesopontine and pontine reticular activity that is associated with the onset of REM sleep. It is also a transmitter of the thalamocortical projection fibers which are responsible for synchronizing cortical activity during non-REM sleep (Pace-Schott and Hobson 2002).

Neuropeptides such as vasoactive intestinal polipeptide (VIP) as well as several hormones are increasingly thought to regulate REM/non-REM cycles (Steiger and Holsboer 1997; Gronfier and Brandenberger 1998). Growth hormone releasing hormone (GHRH) promotes non-REM sleep, while growth hormone (GH) promotes REM sleep. Its metabolite, insulin-like growth factor (IGF-1) promotes wakefulness. Somatostatin reduces the duration of non-REM sleep, but promotes REM sleep, probably by an action within the brainstem. Corticotropin-releasing hormon (CRH, structurally similar to somatostatin) promotes wakefulness and inhibits non-REM sleep. Adrenocorticotropic hormon (ACTH) increases the duration of wakefulness and the lighter stages of non-REM sleep, reduces the duration of stages III and IV of non-REM sleep, and probably has little effect on REM sleep. Glucocorticoids inhibit non-REM sleep. VIP-containing neurons are present in the core of SCN and elsewhere in the hypothalamus. They project to the the median eminence where VIP acts as a releasing factor for prolactin. VIP increases REM sleep, while prolactin promotes it. Oestrogens act in the hypothalamic preoptic area to increase arousal, and inhibit REM sleep.

Nitric oxide (NO) functions primarily as an intercellular messenger that can enhance capillary vasodilation and the synaptic release of neuotransmitters such as acetylcholine. It is produced by mesopontine cholinergic neurons and might help to maintain the cholinergically mediated REM sleep state in the pons and thalamus (Williams et al. 1997). The vascular effects of NO could contribute to the REM-related changes in regional blood flow that are seen in neuroimaging studies (Braun et al. 1997).

Hypocretins (orexins) are peptides located in the synaptic vesicles of neurons in the perifornical area ot the lateral hypothalamus, and tend to stabilize wakefulness and limit the duration of REM sleep (Saper et al. 2001).

Many other substances (e.g. cholecystokinin, insuline, opiod peptides, substance PP, cytokines, prostaglandines, adenosine, etc.) are thought to be involved in the sleep-wake cycle, but their role is more limited or not completely ascertained.

3.4. THE GENETIC REGULATION OF SLEEP

It is now known that the interlocking positive-negative feedback mechanism that controls gene trascription in individual cells of the SCN of the hypothalamus represents the molecular basis of circadian rhythmicity in mammals (Moore and Speh 1993; Liu and Pepper 2000). Circadian rhythmicity emerges from SCN cells by action potentials that impinge in adjacent nuclei of the anterior hypothalamus; these nuclei in turn convey circadian rhythmicity to structures that control rhythmic physiological processes such as sleep, temperature and endocrine output.

Feedback to the SCN circadian oscillator possibly occurs through the secretion of melatonin from the pineal gland. The combined action of positive and negative feedback loops creates a suite of molecular signals that reliably recur at precise times over 24 hours cycles and can be read by cytoplasmic mechanisms in SCN cells and translated into reliably recurring events, such as changes in membrane potentials (Reppert and Weaver 2001). Such signals, in turn, can be transmitted to connecting neurons and, ultimately, to those structures that control physiological processes with circadian rhythmicity. SCN neurons probably synchronize by means of GABA neurotransmission (Miche and Colwell 2001).

3.5. WHAT ARE DREAMS MADE OF?

It is generally accepted, but not ultimately proven, that dreaming is a phenomenon of REM sleep (Takeuchi et al. 2001). Dreams appear to be initiated in REM sleep by pontine centres, particularly the LDT/PPT. These are responsible for muscle atonia and project to the cerebral cortex. According to the original theory of the *"chemical activation-synthesis of dreaming"* (Hobson and McCarley 1977), the brain could work as an effective "dream generator", being able to block, at the level of the pontine structures, the sensorial inputs and, at the same time, to produce internal information, that would then be elaborated by forebrain structures and eventually synthetized as dream experiences.

Subsequently, neuroimaging data obtained from healthy volunteers have allowed the same authors to refine their theory on the genesis of dream experiences. In particular, the interaction between forebrain and brainstem activation in REM sleep, led them to the formulation of the hypothesis of the tridimensional "AIM" (Activation, Input source, Modulation) model of conscious states (Hobson et al. 2000). In this articulated model (see Hobson and Pace Schott 2002 for details), distributed networks of brain structures, and not specific "localized" centres, control waking cognitive skills, perception and consciousness. For example, activation of the forebrain through the brainstem reticular activating system occurs both in REM sleep and in the waking state, but such activation is aminergically deficient and cholinergically driven only in REM sleep. One possible explanation is that during REM sleep, activated thalamic nuclei transmit endogenous cholinergic stimuli that lead to the sensory phemomena of dreaming. The simultaneous activation of medial forebrain structures, especially limbic and paralimbic areas of the cortex and subcortex (including the amygdala), could underlie dream emotionality and the highly social nature of dreaming (Pace-Schott 2001). Strong activation of the basal ganglia might mediate the fictional motion of dreams, as they are extensively connected with REM-regulatory areas in the mesopontine tegmentum (Braun et al. 1997). Deactivation of executive areas in the dorsolateral prefrontal cortex during non-REM sleep might explain the relevant executive deficiencies of dream mentation, including disorientation, illogicity, impaired working memory and amnesia for dreams. Finally, according to this theory, cortical areas located in the medial occipital and temporal lobes generate the visual imagery of dreams. Hobson's theory of dreams focuses on identifying the two chemical systems inside the brain that regulate the waking and the dreaming experience (the "adrenergic" and the "cholinergic" systems). According to Hobson, the interplay of these chemical processes is responsible for all of consciousness, including dreams.

It is likely that mixed non-REM/REM sleep states exist, particularly later in the night (Suzuki et al. 2004). This suggests that REM sleep processes extend into what is conventionally classified as non-REM sleep. However, it is only during REM sleep that real dream experiences appear, with topo-chronological alienity, pluriperceptive vividness of the hallucinatory type, autorappresentation in the dream scene, loss of the sense of reality and of the control of thought course, intense emotional involvement (Bosinelli et al. 1974). During dream mentation, which is associated with REM sleep, there are perceptual phenomena mostly of internal origin, so that REM sleep appears to be associated with some kind of perception and consciousness (Fagioli 2002). It has been proposed that REM sleep has to be somehow regarded as a sort of "third state" of existence, next to wakefulness and slow wave sleep (Coenen 1998).

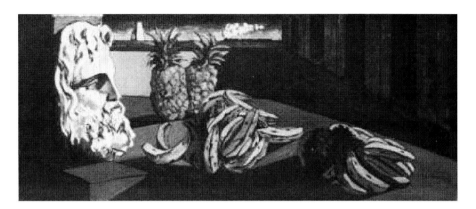

Figure 3.8. "The transformed dream" by Giorgio De Chirico (1913) - Saint Louis, Art Museum.

Finally, the meaning of dreams still remains mysterious, unless we refer to psychoanalytic theories, but this is a matter of great controversy (Hobson 2003) and goes far beyond the aim of this book - see Figure 3.8 for an artistic representation of the meaning of dreams. The interested reader may refer to the paper by Mancia (1983) for a classical and insightful review on the relationships between psychoanalysis and neurophysiology. Quite interestingly, in the same years the Nobel Prize laureate Francis Crick formulated the hypothesis that dreams subserve the process of unlearning, i.e. forgetting or removing superfluous and useless information from the brain storage capacity (Crick and Mitchison 1983). This speculative hypothesis still represents a thought-provoking bridge between psychoanalytic theories and neurobiology.

3.6. PHARMACOLOGICAL MODULATION OF SLEEP

Drugs are often used in the treatment of sleep disorders, either to promote alertness and wakefulness (psychostimulants) or to promote or improve the quality of sleep (hypnotics) (see also Stahl 2000, for an extensive review on pharmacological mechanisms).

3.6.1. Psychostimulants And Wakefulness-Promoting Drugs

The use of CNS stimulants is limited by the risk of abuse potential, withdrawal symptoms, tolerance, side-effects, drug interactions and the dangers of overdose. Apart of caffeine and other xantines (usually self-administered), amphetamines represent the majority of prescribed drugs. They enhance activity at dopamine, noradrenaline and 5HT synapses, with their action being prominent in the brainstem ascending reticular activating system and cerebral cortex. The alerting effect of amphetamines are probably due to noradrenaline or 5HT release or to both of these. The most important single drugs are as follows.

Amphetamine: a racemic mixture of dextro- and levo-amphetamines, has a relatively more central than peripheral action compared to ephedrine but less central action than dexamphetamine.

Dexamphetamine: the dextro-isomer of amphetamine, is three-four time more effective than the levo-isomer.

Metamphetamine: the most rapidly absorbed and effective amphetamine, with a peak blood level reached at 1 hour after ingestion. It is rarely used in clinical settings, and is subject to drug abuse. It is also known as methedrine and "speed".

Methylphenydate: a piperidin derivative structurally similar to amphetamine, blocks dopamine reuptake by binding to the dopamine transporter. It has a similar but less marked effect on noradrenaline and 5HT reuptake (Challman and Lipsky 2000). It is rapidly absorbed and de-esterified to an inactive metabolite, ritalinic acid, in the liver and then excreted in the urine. It acts particularly on the thalamus and on the cerebral cortex, but causes more sympathetic side-effects than amphetamines. It is used to treat attention deficit and hyperactivity disorder and excessive daytime sleepiness (narcolepsy).

Cocaine: subject to drug abuse, it is very similar to methylphenydate in both its structure and its mechanism of action. It potentiates the effects of noradrenaline and adrenaline, thus increasing alertness and motor activity, releasing fatigue and causing euphoria. It reduces total sleep time, increases sleep latency and reduces both stages 3/4 of non-REM sleep and REM sleep (Boutrel and Coob 2004). Cocaine overdose leads to epileptic seizures and delirium, and chronic use causes sleep deprivation. Abrupt withdrawal causes depression and prolonged sleep with REM sleep rebound. Tolerance frequently develops and chronic use is associated with death for cardiac dysrhythmias, myocardial infarction and stroke.

Ecstasy: a hallucinogen chemically related to metamphetamine, NMDA (N-methyl-D-aspartate, an excitotoxic aminoacid), and mescaline. It causes a reduction in REM sleep and its use may be followed by depression.

Altogether, amphetamines reduce total sleep time, increase sleep latency, slightly reduce the duration of stages 3 and 4 of non-REM sleep. On the other hand, they prolong wakefulness, increase the level of alertness, increase confidence, concentration and loquacity, improve psychomotor and mental performances, and lead to euphoria and easy excitability. At times they can possibly lead to agitation and aggression and even to paranoid psychosis, with auditory hallucinations. Depression and fatigue often follow the phase of excitation. Other relevant side effects include peripheral sympathetic and motor symptoms, i.e. rise in body temperature, tachycardia, abdominal spasms, xerostomia, headache and tremor, severe hypertension.

Modafinil (2-((diphenylmethyl)sulphynil)acetamide): this so called "wake promoter" increases the activity of histaminergic neurons in the TMN of the posterior hypothalamus, which promote wakefuness. There is some evidence that this drug inhibits the VLPO by increasing its noradrenergic input, possibly as a result of an increase in locus coeruleus activity (Gallopin et al. 2004). Unlike amphetamines, it does not increase motor activity or have any peripheral sympathetic effect. It is widely used in narcolepsy (US Modafinil in Narcolepsy Multicenter Study Group 2000).

3.6.2. Hypnotics

Hypnotics are drugs used to promote or improve the quality of sleep, and their history began with the bromides first available in 1857, followed by the introduction of barbiturates at the end of 19th century and benzodiazepines (BZ) around 1960. BZ are widely used worldwide, with a stable 8% per year increase, especially in Western countries. There is a great deal of scientific and at times ethical debate on their use and effectiveness, but it is clear that this drug class has represented a milestone in the treatment of insomnia.

The ideal hypnotic drug should promote sleep without causing any residual daytime sleepiness or any other phenomenon related to CNS depression, but to date none of the available drugs owns all these properties in combination.

Barbiturates

Barbiturates are substituted pyrimidine derivatives with a core barbituric acid (a malonic-aldheyde derivative) structure. They act on the GABA-A receptor complex (Figure 3.9) at a site close but different from the target of BZ.

The GABA-A receptor consists of a GABA binding site on the cell membrane close to the chloride channels, which are opened by GABA, so that the post-synaptic membrane becomes hyperpolarized. This inhibits the activity of neurons and reduces their frequency of firing. Barbiturates have a widespread action in the CNS, but particularly in the midbrain reticular formation, and cause generalized CNS depression. The individual drugs are represented by amobarbital, butobarbital and secobarbital. They reduce sleep latency and the duration of REM sleep. The duration of stage 2 of non-REM sleep is increased, but stages 3 and 4 of non-REM sleep become shorter and the number of arousals is reduced. They may cause sedation, anaesthesia and even death in case of overdosage. Abrupt withdrawal leads to REM sleep rebound or convulsive seizures. Daytime sedation is common, because of the long duration of action (6-8 hours). They are also used as muscle relaxants and may cause severe dose-dependent respiratory depression.

Benzodiazepines

Benzodiazepines (BZ) contain a benzene ring linked to a seven member diazepine ring. Most of them show GABAergic mechanisms of action, interacting with the GABA-A receptor. BZ bind to this macromolecular GABA receptor chloride ionophore complex close to the GABA binding site and at a location close to, but distinct from the binding sites of barbiturates, alcohol and chloral. Other hypnotics, like zopiclon, zolpidem and zaleplon bind to different receptor sites (see below). The action of BZ on the GABA receptor complex is most marked in the hypothalamus, thalamus and limbic system, and this explains the sedative and hypnotic effects of BZ as well as their anxiolytic, muscle relaxant and antiepileptic actions. Subtypes of the BZ receptors have been identified (i.e. BZ1, omega-1; BZ2, omega-2) but their significance remains unclear. BZ in low dose have a sedative effect and at a higher dose induce sleep, and may even lead to coma. They reduce spontaneous activity and response to afferent stimuli of the ascending reticular activating system and block the EEG responses that are evoked by stimulation. The EEG during wakefulness shows a reduction and slowing of the alpha rhythm with an increase in the beta rhythm, particularly in the frontal cortex. BZ increase total sleep time, shorten sleep latency, reduce the number of awakenings and provide a sense of deep and refreshing sleep. REM sleep latency is prolonged and the duration of REM sleep is reduced. There are fewer eye movements and less dreaming during REM sleep, except with short-acting drugs, such as triazolam, which cause a rebound in REM sleep late in the night. Daytime sedation (*"hangover"* effect) is more prominent with long-acting drugs, such as flurazepam (Table 3.2). Tolerance is common, and abrut withdrawal may lead to a specific syndrome characterized by disrupted sleep, vivid dreams and nightmares, associated with an increase in REM sleep and in stages 3 and 4 of non-REM sleep (Gillin 1991).

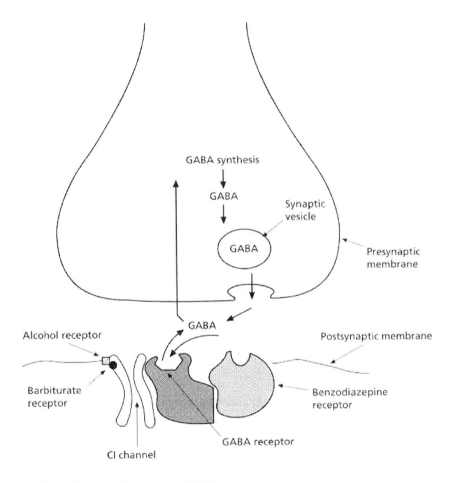

Figure 3.9. Action of hypnotic drugs at the GABA-A receptor.

Other Hypnotic Drugs

- Zopiclone is a cyclopirrolone and binds to the GABA-A receptor complex at a different site to BZ. It does not influence REM sleep, but reduces the stage 1 of non-REM sleep and the number of arousals. It is short-acting but can cause daytime sedation, with similar anxiolytic, muscle relaxant and anticonvulsant action to BZ.

Table 3.2. Most common benzodiazepines and their effect on sleep

Drug	Effect on sleep
Alprazolam	Long acting
Clonazepam*	Long acting
Clorazepate	Long acting
Diazepam**	Short acting
Flunitrazepam	Short acting
Flurazepam	Intermediate to long acting
Lorazepam**	Long acting
Lormetazepam	Intermediate
Midazolam	Very short acting
Nitrazepam	Intermediate to long acting
Oxazepam	Intermediate
Triazolam	Short acting

* = Mainly used as anticonvulsant.
** = Also used as anticonvulsant.

- Zolpidem is a imidazolpyridine derivative chemically not related to BZ, and acting at the GABA-A receptor complex close to, but at a different site from BZ. It has little effect on sleep architecture and is not anxiolytic, muscle relaxant or anticonvulsant.
- Zaleplon is a pyrazopyrimidine compound, binding to BZ1 (omega-1) receptors, in a similar manner to zolpidem. It has a dose-related effect in reducing sleep latency, but it does not increase total sleep time because of its short duration of action. It is anxiolytic with muscle relaxant action.
- Alcohol: although it cannot be defined a drug *sensu stricto*, ethyl alcohol (ethanol) surely represents the oldest millenary "natural" compound used by man for its anxiolityc, euphorizing and hypnotic effects. It acts on the GABA receptor complex in a way similar to BZ, but at a slightly different site, and it is also a glutamate inhibitor. It influences particularly the reticular activating formation and causes generalized CNS depression. It is anxiolityc and weakly hypnotic, reducing the total sleep time and sleep latency. It also reduces the latencies before stages 3 and 4 of non-REM sleep, increases their duration, and suppresses REM sleep. It has a short duration of action, so that as the blood alcohol level falls during the night REM sleep rebound occurs, with vivid dreams, loss of non-REM sleep and frequent awakenings. Chronic ingestion leads to the disruption of the sleep-wake cycle, up to the complete disintegration of sleep architecture, as tolerance develops and the quantity of alcohol assumption progressively increases. Sedation is common and respiratory depression may frequently occur.
- Melatonin, N-5-methoxy-N-acetyl-tryptamine, is synthetized from tryptophan after it has been converted to serotonin (Brzezinski 1997). A small amount of melatonin is stored in the pineal gland, but it is synthetized and secreted in pulses in response to noradrenaline release at synapses within the pineal gland. It is a physiological marker of the circadian function, but it also acts as a hormone of darkness to

reinforce the synchronization of sleep with the dark-light cycle of the environment. The pineal gland acts a transducer, converting a photo-period signal into a chemical signal. Melatonin has a soporific effect which is greatest during the day and probably mediated by activation of inhibitory GABAergic neurons, possibly through the actions of cytokines. It does not seem to alter the proportions of non-REM and REM sleep, but if given during the day it usually promotes stages 1 and 2 of non-REM sleep.

3.7. THE NEUROIMAGING OF SLEEP

More detailed explorations of sleep in humans are now accessible to experimental challenges using positron emission tomography (PET) and other neuroimaging techniques. During the last few years, functional imaging studies using PET have yielded original data on the functional neuroanatomy of human sleep. The published PET data describe a very reproducible functional neuroanatomy of sleep, with a marked decrease of cerebral blood flow signal across thalami and fronto-parietal association cortices.

During non-REM sleep, significant regional declines in glucose or oxygen consumption have been demonstrated in the pons, thalamus, hypothalamus, caudate nucleus, lateral and medial regions of the prefrontal cortex. On the other hand, during REM sleep blood flow increases have been observed in the pons, midbrain, thalamus, amygdala, hypothalamus, and basal ganglia (Braun et al. 1997). In REM sleep there is a relative deactivation of the dorsolateral prefrontal cortex, while activation of limbic and paralimbic regions of the forebrain is increased (Maquet 1996). Frontal deactivations have also been described by functional magnetic resonance imaging (fMRI) studies of REM sleep (e.g. Lovblad et al. 1999).

Moreover, the posteromedial aspect of the parietal lobe (precuneus, posterior cingulate, and retrosplenial cortices), along with lateral parietal and prefrontal cortices, were found to be significantly less active than the rest of the brain during both slow wave (non-REM) sleep (Maquet et al. 1997; Andersson et al. 1998), and REM sleep (Maquet et al. 1996; Braun et al. 1997). The interpretation of this selective deactivation is uncertain. Moreover, it has been shown that the precuneus belongs to a fronto-parietal associative network which is particularly active during conscious wakefulness (Cavanna and Trimble 2006). Since impaired consciousness of the self and its environment represents a key feature shared by the different sleep stages, the abovementioned results of functional neuroimaging studies might provide further evidence for an active participation of these brain areas in conscious processes (Maquet et al. 1999). In particular, these data fit well with the recently proposed hypothesis that the precuneate cortex, which is characterized by widespread cortical and subcortical connections, can play a central role in the neural network correlates of consciousness (Cavanna and Trimble 2006).

3.8. SLEEP DISORDERS

Insomnia is the most frequent sleep disorder, although several kinds of pathological impairments of consciousness may occur during sleep or excessive daytime sleepiness. Sleep disorders are classified according to the following subgroups (American Academy of Sleep Medicine 2005): 1) insomnias, 2) sleep related breathing disorders, 3) hypersomnias of central origin, 4) circadian rhythm sleep disorders, 5) parasomnias (i.e. sleep-associated disorders), 6) sleep related movement disorders, 7) isolated symptoms and unresolved issues, 8) sleep disorders not otherwise specified. In this paragraph we will mainly focus on hypersomnias and sleep-related movement disorders, for their relevance to the field of consciousness studies.

3.8.1. Hypersomnias

Hypersomnias are characterized by unrefreshing sleep at night leading to either a prolonged daytime sleep episode or a persistent need to sleep during the day. Narcolepsy, which is usually included in this group, is a chronic neurologic disorder affecting sleep regulation and causing excessive sleepiness and, in most cases, cataplexy. The latter refers to partial or generalised, almost invariably bilateral, brief attacks (less than 1 minute) of loss of skeletal muscle tone, triggered by emotional stimuli (usually amusement, power and elation) (Overeen et al. 2001; Zeman et al. 2004). Generalised attacks can lead to dangerous collapse, with awareness usually preserved. Other common symptoms include sleep paralysis (inability to move for a few minutes at the beginning or end of sleep); hypnagogic hallucinations (vivid, dream-like experiences at sleep onset); disturbed nocturnal sleep pattern, associated with an increased rate of behavioral abnormalities in sleep, such as sleep-walking and automatic behaviors. In the early 1960s it was shown that narcolepsy is primarily a REM sleep disorder: people with narcolepsy enter REM sleep more quickly than usual when they fall asleep, and the associated symptoms (including cataplexy) all represent intrusions of REM sleep phenomena (muscular atonia and dream imagery) into wakefulness (Rechstchaffen et al. 1963). Later on, it was docovered that many people with narcolepsy share the tissue antigen type HLA DR2 (Juji et al. 1984), thus suggesting that narcolepsy can be the consequence of an autommune process, which results in destruction of hypocretin-producing cells. Although this theory is still controversial (Mignot 2000), the involvment of hypocretin in narcolepsy, has been confirmed by the finding that doberman dogs can have familial narcolepsy associated with a gene mutation causing a deletion of the hypocretin type 2 receptor (Lin et al. 1999). Furthermore, hypocretin concentrations were markedly reduced in the cerebrospinal fluid of patients with narcolepsy associated with cataplexy (Nishino 2000), and in the brains from patients with narcolepsy examined at autopsy (Peyron et al. 2000; Thannickal et al. 2000).

3.8.2. Sleep-Related Movement Disorders

During sleep, movement is largely decreased, due to the greater inhibition of lower motor neuron activity, especially in postural muscles during REM sleep. Motor activity can break through either if central activity increases or if its inhibition fails even transiently. This is the main reason why there are fewer motor disorders in REM sleep than in non-REM sleep, with the exception of "REM sleep behavior disorder", in which release of motor inhibition allows complex movements, reflecting the content of vivid dreams, to be enacted. Several sleep motor disorders are known, but we will shortly describe here only epilepsy, sleep paralysis, sleep walking and REM sleep behavioral disorder, focusing on their impact on the normal conscious state.

Epilepsy

Epilepsy belongs to this class of disorders, as sleep and the transition to wakefulness affect the threshold for electrical epileptic discharges to arise and propagate. Epileptic seizures occur particularly at arousal or during a sleep phase transition, and any factor which increases non-REM sleep tends to precipitate epilepsy. Nocturnal epilepsy is characterized by seizures occurring either early in the night (stages 1 and 2 of non-REM sleep (Minecan et al. 2002) or 1-2 hours after the transition from sleep to wakefulness in the morning. The most common types of epilepsy (generalized epilepsy, temporal lobe epilepsy, frontal lobe epilepsy etc.) are all somehow related to sleep (Mahowald and Schenck 1997). The relationship between epilepsy and consciousness will be the subject of chapter 5.

Sleep Paralysis

Sleep paralysis is the inability to move at the onset or end of sleep while the subject is awake. It is also called "Ondine's curse", after the name of the nymph of a traditional Scandinavian myth, main character of Jean Giraudox's drama "Ondine" (1939). In this drama, the hero, guilty of betraying the nymph, is condemned to lose all his automatic movements.

Sleep paralysis is often triggered by sleep deprivation, irregular sleep-wake patterns or psychological stress. There is full awareness of the situation, which is usually frightening.

Sleep Walking

Sleep walking (*somnambulism*) is a common manifestation of incomplete arousal from stages 3 and 4 of non-REM sleep in children and young adults, and usually occurs in the first third of the night. Subjects may sit up in bed, open the eyes, move around almost purposefully, often avoding obstacles (Kavey et al. 1990). Noisy sleep environment, distended bladder, pain, stress, fever or obstructive sleep apnoeas may all precipitate sleep walking in susceptible subjects.

REM Sleep Behavior Disorder

REM sleep behavior disorder (RBD): the essential features are vivid, aggressive dreams associated with abnormal movements in REM sleep (Schenck et al. 2002). These are due to abnormal REM sleep generation in the pons and loss of the normal atonia of REM sleep. It may be caused acutely by drug intoxication (e.g. alcohol, amphetamine, cocaine, etc.) or be present in chronic neurological disorders, such as extrapyramidal disorders, Alzheimer's disease, Creuzfeldt-Jakob's disease, and narcolepsy.

In RBD dreams are often quite vivid (usually threatening), with accompanying abnormal limb and trunk movements occurring most commonly during the first REM sleep cycle. More complex, organized movements appear as the condition becomes more severe: finger ponting, laughing, shouting, getting out of bed, and aggressive behaviors are not uncommon. "Status dissociatus" may represent a severe form of RBD, with a continuous dissociation of non-REM and REM sleep features as shown by the EEG, with rapid oscillations of sleep states, and features of wakefulness (Mahowald and Schenck 1991).

3.9. SLEEP AND THE CONSCIOUS BRAIN

Despite the fact that sleep covers one third of human lifetime and the amount of scientific research on sleep and its disorders, we are still far from a full understanding of the functional meaning of this physiological phenomenon. It is commonly believed that non-REM sleep, especially in its delta wave component, is correlated with the preservation and restoration of basic vegetative functions, whereas REM sleep seems to be mainly correlated to higher cerebral and mental functions. In particular, delta wave non-REM sleep might have a relationship, possibly regulated by an instinctive situation, with the preceding state of wakefulness and with its correlated metabolic, thermoregulatory and homeostatic needs (McGinty and Szymusiak 1990). Sleep may also have a biochemical compensatory function toward wakefulness, since overall neuronal glucose utilization is higher during wakefulness, while the process is reversed during sleep, so that glucose can be available for neuronal activity during the following wakefulness period (Buchsbaum et al. 2001). On the other hand, REM sleep may absolve the primary function of brain restoration and cortical maturation. This phase is therefore deeply involved in psychological functions and in the development of specific mental activities. REM sleep processing and integration of newly acquired information into existing neural "templates" enables future responses to reflect previous experiences of the individual and inherited potentials. REM sleep may also play a neurodevolpmental role, as it is most prolonged in the mammals whose offspring are least mature at birth, and in neonates and young children (Jouvet 1998).

Interactions between the neocortex and hippocampus during sleep might promote the storage and consolidation of information acquired during previous waking states (Buzsàki 1996). Cortically consolidated memories originally stored during non-REM sleep by iterative processes, such as information outflow from the hippocampus, would thus be integrated with other stored memories during REM sleep. Consequently, dreaming would represent the conscious experience of hyperperassociative brain activation, that is maximal in REM sleep. This hypothesis, already adumbrated by Hartley as early as in 1791, is consistent with the idea that "normal" associations are loosened during REM sleep and such loosening is linked to the bizarreness of dream experiences (Hobson et al. 1987).

Both REM and non-REM sleep appear to be involved in memory consolidation, but in different ways (Cipolli et al. 2004). Recall of cognitive procedures works better if there is a sequence of non-REM and then REM sleep phases, but declarative memory does not appear to require REM sleep (Smith 2001), and may be related to spinal activity in stage 2 of non-REM sleep (Schabus et al. 2004). As a result of several studies on sleep-dependent memory consolidation processes, the importance of sleep-dependent changes for brain plasticity is becoming more widely recognized (Stickgold et al. 2001).

The impaired ability to integrate information among specialized thalamocortical modules – a proposed theoretical requirement for consciousness (Tononi 2004) – may underlie the fading of consciousness in non-REM sleep early in the night. Transcranial magnetic stimulation and high-density EEG techcniques have recently demonstrated the widespread breakdown of cortical effective connectivity (the ability of cortical areas to interact effectively) during sleep (Massimini et al. 2005).

In conclusion, the complex interactions between the brainstem reticular formation and nonspecific diencephalic nuclei represent the neurobiological (i.e., neuroanatomical, neurochemical and neurophysiological) substrate for sleep-induced alterations of consciousness, and this system acts, using a musical metaphor, as the conductor of the so-called "neural orchestra" which plays the sleep suite (Coenen et al. 1998). Within this metaphor, consciousness might be the music, coming out as the "free", and hence personal and somehow artistic, expression of a huge population of neurons firing in the tonic mode.

3.10. REFERENCES

American Academy of Sleep Medicine. *International classification of sleep disorders. Diagnostic and coding manual, 2nd edition.* American Academy of Sleep Medicine, Westchester, Illinois 2005.

Andersson JLR, Onoe H, Hetta J, Lindstrom K, Valind S, Lilja A, Sundin A, Fasth KJ, Westerberg G, Broman JE, Watanabe Y, Langstrom B. Brain networks affected by synchronized sleep visualized by positron emission tomography. *J Cereb Blood Flow Metab.* 1998;18:701-715.

Batini C, Moruggi G, Palestrini M, Rossi CF, Zanchetti A. Effects of complete pontine transection on the sleep wakefulness-rhythm: the midpontine pretrigeminal preparation. *Arch Ital Biol.* 1959;96:1-12.

Bentivoglio M, Steriade M. Brainstem-diencephalic circuits as a structural substrate of the ascendent reticular activation concept. In: Mancia M, Marini M eds. *The diencephalon and sleep.* Raven Press, New York 1990:7-29.

Bosinelli M, Cicogna P, Molinari S. The tonic-phase model and the feeling of self-partecipation in different stages of sleep. *Ital J Psychol.* 1974; 1: 35-75

Boutrel B, Koob GF. What keeps us awake: the neuropharmacology of stimulants and wakefulness promoting medications. *Sleep.* 2004;27:1181-1194.

Braun AR, Balkin TJ, Wesenten NJ, Carson RE, Varga M, Baldwin P, Selbie S, Belenky G, Herscovitch P. Regional cerebral blood flow throughout the sleep-wake cycle: an (H2O)-O15 PET study. *Brain.* 1997;120:173-197.

Brzezinski A. Melatonin in humans. *N Engl J Med.* 1997;336:186-195.

Buchsbaum MS,Hazlett EA,Wu J,Bunney WA. Positron emission tomography with deoxyglucose F18 imaging of sleep. *Neuropsychopharmacology.* 2001; 25: S50-S56.

Buzsàki G. The hippocampo-neocortical dialogue. *Cereb Cortex.* 1996;6: 81-92.

Cavanna AE, Trimble MR. The precuneus: a review of its functional anatomy and behavioural correlates. *Brain.* 2006;129:564-583.

Challman TD, Lipsky JJ. Methylphenidate: its pharmacology and use. *Mayo Clin Proc.* 2000;73: 711-721.

Chokroverty S. *Sleep disorder*. Philadelphia: Butterworth 1999.

Cipolli C, Fagioli I, Mazzetti M, Tozzi G. Incorporation of presleep stimuli and dream contents: evidence for a consolidation effect on declarative knowledge during REM sleep? *J Sleep Res.* 2004;13:317-326.

Coenen AML. Neuronal phenomena associated with vigilance and consciousness: from cellular mechanisms to electroencephalographic patterns. *Conscious Cogn.* 1998;7:42-53.

Cordeau JP, Mancia M. Effects of an electroencephalographic synchronization mechanism originating in the lower brainstem. *Electroenceph Clin Neurophysiol.* 1959;11:551-564.

Crick F, Mitchison G. The function of dream sleep. *Nature.* 1983;304:111.

Douglas NJ. The sleepy patient. *J Neurol Neurosurg Psychiatry.* 2001;71 (Suppl I):13-16.

Espana RA, Scammell TE. Sleep neurobiology for the clinician. *Sleep* 2004; 27: 811-820.

Fagioli I. Mental activity during sleep. *Sleep Med Res.* 2002; 6:307-320.

Gallopin T, Luppi P-H, Rambert FA, Frydman A, Forr P. Effect of the wake-promoting agent modafinil on sleep-promoting neurons from the ventrolateral preoptic nucleus: an in vitro pharmacologic study. *Sleep.* 2004;27:19-25.

Gillin JC. The long and the short of sleeping pills. *N Engl J Med.* 1991;324: 1735-1736.

Gronfier C, Brandenberger G. Ultradian rhythms in primary and adrenal hormones: their relations to sleep. *Sleep Med Res.* 1996;2:17-29.

Hartley D. *Observations on man, his frame, his duty and his expectations*. Johnson, London 1791.

Hobson JA. *Dreaming: an introduction to the science of sleep*. Oxford University Press, Oxford 2003.

Hobson JA, McCarley R, Wyzinki PW. Sleep cycle reciprocal oscillation discharge by two brainstem neuronal groups. *Science.* 1975;189:55-58.

Hobson JA, McCarley RW. The brain as a dream generator: an activation synthesis. Hypothesis of the dream process. *Am J Psychiatry.* 1977;134: 1335-1348.

Hobson JA, Hoffman E, Helfand R, Kostner D. Dream bizarreness and the activation-synthesis hypothesis. *Human Neurobiol.* 1987;6:157-164.

Hobson JA, Pace-Schott EF, Stickgold R. Dreaming and the brain: toward a cognitive neuroscience of conscious states. *Behav Brain Sci.* 2000;23:793-842.

Hobson JA, Pace Schott EF. The cognitive neuroscience of sleep: neuronal systems, consciousness and learning. *Nature Rev Neurosci.* 2002;3:679-693.

Huguenard JR. Anatomical and physiological considerations in thalamic rhythm generation. *J Sleep Res.* 1998;7(Suppl 1):24-29.

Jouvet M. Paradoxical sleep as a programming system. *J Sleep Res.* 1998; 7:1-5.

Jujii T, Satake M, Honda Y, Doi Y. HLA antigens in Japanese patients with narcolepsy: all the patients were DR2 positive. *Tissue Antigen.* 1984;24:316-319.

Kavey NB, Whyte J, Resor SR, Gidro-Frank S. Somnambulism in adults. *Neurology.* 1990; 40:749-752.

Kryger MH, Roth T, Dement WC eds. *Principles and practice of sleep medicine.* Saunders, Philadelphia 2000.

Leonard CS, Linas R. Serotoninergic and cholinergic inhibition of mesopontine cholinergic neurons controlling REM sleep: an in vitro electrophysiological study. *Neuroscience.* 1994;59:309-330.

Lin L, Faraco J, Li R, Kadotani H, Rogers W, Lin X, Qiu X, De Jong PJ, Nishino S, Mignot E. The sleep disorder canine narcolepsy is caused by a mutation in the hypocretin (orexin) receptor 2 gene. *Cell.* 1999;98:365-376.

Liu C, Reppert SM. GABA synchronizes clock cells within the suprachiasmatic circadian clock. *Neuron.* 2000;25:123-128.

Lovblad K.O. Silent functional magnetic resonance imaging demonstrates focal activation in rapid eye movement sleep. *Neurology.* 1999;53;2193-2195.

Mahowald MW, Schenck CK. Sleep disorders. In: Engel J, Pedley T eds. *Epilepsy: a comprehensive textbook.* Lippincott-Raven, Philadelphia 1997: 2705-2715.

Mahowald MW, Schenck CH. Status dissociatus: a perspective on states of being. *Sleep.* 1991;14:69-79.

Mancia M. Archaeology of Freudian thought and the history of neurophysiology. *Int J Psychoanal.* 1983; 10:185-192.

Maquet P, Peters J, Aerts J, Delfiore G, Degueldre C, Luxen A, Functional neuroanatomy of human REM sleep and dreaming. *Nature.* 1996; 383: 163-166.

Maquet P, Degueldre C, Delfiore G, Aerts J, Peters JM, Luxen A,Franck G. Functional neuroanatomy of human slow wave sleep. *J Neurosci.* 1997;17: 2807-2812.

Maquet P, Faymonville ME, Degueldre C, Delfiore G, Franck G, Luxen A, Lamy M. Functional neuroanatomy of hypnotic state. *Biol Psychiatry.* 1999; 45:327-333.

Massimini M, Ferrarelli F, Huber R, Esser SK, Singh H, Tononi G. Breakdown of cortical effective connectivity during sleep. *Science* 2005;309: 2228-2232.

McGinty DJ, Szymusiak RS. *Hypothalamic thermoregulatory control of slow wave sleep.* In: Mancia M, Marini G eds. The diencephalon and sleep. Raven Press, New York 1990, 97-110.

Miche S, Colwell CS. Cellular communication and coupling within the suprachiasmatic nucleus. *Chronobiol Int.* 2001;18: 579-600.

Mignot E. Perspectives in narcolepsy and hypocretin (orexin) research.*Sleep Med.* 2000;1: 87-90.

Mignot E, Lammers GJ, Ripley B, Okun M, Nevsimalova S, Overeen S. The role of cerebrospinal fluid hypocretin measurement in the diagnosis of narcolepsy and other hypersomnias. *Arch Neurol.* 2002; 59:1553-1562.

Minecan D, Natarajan A, Marzec M, Malow B. Relationship of epileptic seizures to sleep stage and sleep depth. *Sleep* 2002;25: 899-904.

Moore R, Speh JC. GABA in the mammalian suprachiasmatic nucleus and its role in the diurnal rhythmicity. *Nature.* 1993;387:596-603.

Moruzzi G, Magoun HW. Brainstem reticular formation and activation of the EEG. *Electroenceph Clin Neurophysiol*. 1949; 1:455-473.

Nishino S, Ripley B, Ovreen S, Lammers GJ, Mignon E. Hypocretin (orexin) deficiency in human narcolepsy. *Lancet*. 2000;355:39-40.

Nitz D, Siegel JM. GABA release in the locus coeruleus as a function of sleep-wake state. *Neuroscience*. 1997a;78:795-801.

Nitz D, Siegel JM. GABA release in the dorsal raphe nucleus: role in the control of REM sleep. *Am J Physiol*. 1997b; 273: R451-R455.

Overeen S, Mignon E, van Dijik JG, Lammers GJ. Narcolepsy: clinical features, new physiological insights and future perspectives. *J Clin Neurophysiol*. 2001;18:78-105.

Pace Schott EF. "Theory of mind", social cognition and dreaming. *Sleep Res Soc Bull*. 2001;7;33-36.

Pace-Schott EF, Hobson JA. The neurobiology of sleep: genetics, cellular physiology and subcortical networks. *Nature Rev Neurosci*. 2002;3:591-605.

Peyron C, Farmaco J, Rogers W, Ripley B, Overeen S, Charnay Y, Nevsimalova S, Aldrich M, Reynolds D, Albin R, Li R, Hungs M, Pedrazzoli M, Padigaru M, Kucherlapati M, Fan J, Maki R, Lammers JG, Bouras C, Kucherlapati R, Nishino S, Mignot E. A mutation in a case of early-onset narcolepsy and a generalised absence of hypocretin peptides in human narcoleptic brains. *Nature Med*. 2000;6:991-997.

Rechtschaffen A, Wolpert E, Dement WC, Mitchell SA, Fisher C. Nocturnal sleep of narcoleptics. *Electroenceph Clin Neurophysiol*. 1963;15:599-609.

Reinoso-Suarez F, Andes I, Rodrigo-Angulo ML, Garzon M. Brain structures and mechanisms involved in the generation of REM sleep. *Sleep Med Res*. 2001;5:63-77.

Reppert SM, Weaver DR. Molecular analysis of mammalian circadian rhythms. *Annu Rev Physiol*. 2001;63:647-676.

Russell N, Gelder V. Recent insights into mammalian circadian rhythms. *Sleep*. 2004;27:166-171.

Saper CB, Chou TC, Scammell TE. The sleep switch hypothalamic control of sleep and wakefulness. *Trends Neurosci*. 200;24:726-731.

Schabus M, Gruber G, Parapatics S, Sauter C, Klosch G, Anderei P, Klimesh W, Saletu B, Zeithofer J. Sleep spindles and their significance for declarative memory consolidation. *Sleep*. 2004;27:1479-1485.

Schenck CH, Mahowald MW. REM sleep behavior disorder: clinical developmental and neuroscience perspectives 16 years after its formal identification in sleep. *Sleep*. 2002;25:120-138.

Sherin JE, Shiromani PJ, McCarley RW, Saper CB. Activation of ventrolateral preoptic neurons during sleep. *Science*. 1996;276:216-219.

Shneerson JM. *Sleep medicine. A guide to sleep and its disorders*. 2nd Edition Blackwell Pub, Malden 2005.

Stahl SM. *Essential psychoparmacology. Neuroscientific basis and practical applications*. 2nd Ed. Cambridge, Cambridge Univesity Press, 2000.

Suzuki H, Uchiyama M, Tagaya H, Ozaki A, Kariyama K, Aritake S, Shibui K, Tan X, Kamei Y, Kuga R. Dreaming during non rapid eye movement sleep in the absence of prior eye movement sleep. *Sleep*. 2004;27:1486-1490.

Smith C. Sleep states and memory processes in humans: procedural versus declarative memory consolidation. *Sleep Med Res.* 2001;5:491-506.

Stickgold R, Hobson JA, Fosse R, Fosse M. Sleep, learning and dream; off-line memory reprocessing. *Science.* 2001;294:1052-1057.

Thannickal TC, Moore RY, Nienhuls R, Ramanathan L, Gulyani S, Aldrich M, Cornford M, Siegel JM. Reduced numbers of hypocretin neurons in human narcolepsy. *Neuron.* 2000;27:469-474.

Tononi G. An information integration theory of consciousness. *BioMed Central Neurosci.* 2004:5:42.

US Modafinil in Narcolepsy Multicenter Study Group: Randomized trial of modafinil as a treatment for excessive daytime somnolence of narcolepsy. *Neurology.* 2000;54:166-175.

Vazquez J, Baghdoyan HA. Basal forebrain acetylcholine release during REMsleep is significantly greater than during waking. *Am J Physiol Reg Integr Comp Physiol.* 2001;280: R598-601.

Williams JA. Vincent SR, Reiner PB. Nitric oxide in rat thalamus changes with behavioural states, local depolarization and brainstem stimulation. *J Neurosci.* 1997;17:420-427.

Zeman A, Britton T, Douglas N, Hsnsen A, Hicks J, Howard R, Meredith A, Smith A, Stores G, Zaiwalla Z. Narcolepsy and excessive daytime sleepiness. *Br Med J.* 2004;329:724-728.

COMA AND DRUG-INDUCED ANESTHESIA

Or when, under ether,
the mind is conscious
but conscious of nothing.

T.S. Eliot, East Coker, from The Four Quartets (1946)

4.1. THE UNRESPONSIVE PATIENT

Progress in intensive care over the last decades has led to an increase in the number of patients who survive severe acute brain damage. An accurate and reliable assessment of the arousal and awareness of consciousness in patients with severe brain damage is of greatest importance for their management and prognosis. Although most of these patients recover from coma within the first days after the injury, some permanently lose all brainstem function (brain death), whereas others progress to "wakeful unawareness" (vegetative state). Moreover, those who recover typically progress through different stages (e.g. minimally conscious state) before fully or partly recovering consciousness. Clinical practice has shown the challenges of identifying signs of these patients' conscious state, which entail perception of the environment and of themselves. Bedside assessment of residual brain function and consciousness in patients who are severely brain-damaged is difficult because motor and verbal responses may be quite limited. In addition, the clinical assessment of consciousness relies on inferences made from responses to external stimuli that are observed at the time of the examination (Wade and Johnston 1999). The first section of this chapter reviews the main clinical notions of altered states of consciousness after severe brain damage, defines bedside assessment of consciousness, and discusses recent functional neuroimaging findings in patients with these disorders. The second part of the chapter will deal with drug-induced anesthesia and how it affects consciousness in otherwise healthy subjects. In particular, it will focus on the neural correlates of loss and recovery of consciousness as outlined by recent functional neuroimaging investigations.

4.2. WHAT CAUSES COMA?

It is crucial to evaluate unresponsive patients from both the diagnostic and prognostic perspective. Knowledge of the anatomical basis of coma is essential for competent evaluation, but must be combined with an understanding of the different, often multi-factorial, medical conditions that can result in impaired consciousness. from an operational perspective, consciousness can be defined as a state of awareness of self and the environment. This state is determined by two separate functions, namely awareness (content of consciousness) and arousal (level of consciousness). These are dependant upon separate physiological and anatomical systems. Clinicopathological correlations coupled with neurophysiological and neuroimaging data have shown that coma is caused by diffuse bilateral hemisphere damage, failure of the brainstem ascending reticular activating system, or both.

Unilateral hemispheric lesions will not result in coma unless there is secondary brain stem compression, caused by herniation, compromising the ascending reticular activating system, a core of grey matter continuous caudally with the reticular intermediate grey lamina of the spinal cord and rostrally with the subthalamus, hypothalamus, and thalamic nuclei. On the other hand, extensive bilateral disturbance of the hemisphere function is required to produce coma. Bilateral thalamic and hypothalamic lesions also cause coma by interrupting activation of the cortex mediated through these structures. A typical magnetic resonance imaging picture of a patient with bilateral ischemic thalamic lesions is shown in Figure 4.1.

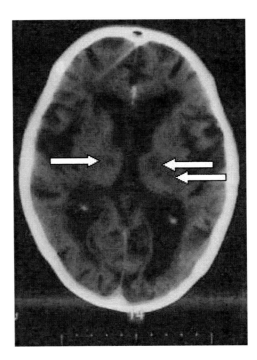

Figure 4.1. Brain MRI scan of a 67 years old woman with bilateral ischemic lesions, involving the anterior and dorsal parts of the right thalamus and the whole left thalamus (white arrows).

The speed of onset, site, and size of a brainstem lesion determine whether it results in coma, therefore brainstem infarction or haemorrhage often causes coma while other brain stem conditions such as multiple sclerosis or tumour rarely do so. Lesions below the level of the pons do not normally result in coma. Drugs and metabolic disease produce coma by a depression of both cortex and ascending reticular activating system function.

Overall, the causes of coma by anatomical site can be divided into:

- diffuse or extensive processes affecting the whole brain;
- supratentorial mass lesions causing tentorial herniation with brain stem compression (associated with other neurological signs such as third nerve palsy and crossed hemiparesis);
- brain stem lesions: for example, compression from posterior fossa mass lesions such as cerebellar haemorrhage/infarction and disorders primarily affecting the brain stem (e.g. basilar artery thrombosis).

In a large study of patients presenting with "medical coma" cerebrovascular disease accounted for 50%, hypoxic ischaemic injury 20%, and various metabolic and infective encephalopathies the remainder (Levy et al. 1981).

4.3. COMA – AND BEYOND

4.3.1. Brain Death

Brain death is defined by the absence of any clinical and neurophysiological sign of brain activity. The concept of brain death as the death of the individual is largely accepted. Moreover, the diagnosis of irreversible loss of brain stem function is now considered as being synonymous with brain death. Quite interestingly, the concept of brainstem death arose a few decades ago from the effectiveness of cardiopulmonary resuscitation. Since the functions of circulation and ventilation could be performed artificially, it become important to identify those patients who were not capable of supporting a sentient life independently.

Brainstem death is established by the following criteria (Medical Consultants on the Diagnosis of Death 1981):

- The cause of coma must be ascertained and it must be known that the patient is suffering from irremediable structural brain damage.

- All complicating factors such as drug intoxication, metabolic unbalances and hypothermia shall have been corrected or excluded.

- The loss of all brainstem reflexes and the demonstration of continuing apnoea in a persistently comatose patient must be ascertained.

4.3.2. Coma

The main feature of coma is the absence of arousal and thus also of any content of consciousness. Coma is a pathological state of eyes-closed unconsciousness from which patients cannot be aroused to wakefulness by stimuli, and have no awareness of self and surroundings (Plum and Posner 1983).

It can be caused by a structural, metabolic, or toxic disturbance of the reticular system and its thalamic projections(Vigand and Vigand 2000).

To be clearly distinguished from syncope, concussion, or other states of transient unconsciousness, coma must persist for at least one hour. However, true coma rarely persists for longer than a month in the absence of complicating metabolic, infectious, or toxic factors. In general, comatose patients who survive begin to awaken and recover gradually within 2-4 weeks. In most survivors of comas who do not spontaneously achieve awareness, coma usually progresses to a a vegetative state or minimally conscious state, or there may be brief or prolonged stages before more complete recovery of consciousness (Vigand and Vigand 2000)

4.3.3. Vegetative State

Bryan Jennett and Fred Plum coined the term "persistent vegetative state" in a classic 1972 article in *The Lancet*. They cited the Oxford English Dictionary to explain their choice of the adjective "vegetative"; to vegetate means to "live merely a physical life devoid of intellectual activity or social intercourse" and vegetative describes "an organic body capable of growth and development but devoid of sensation and thought". Persistent vegetative state has been defined as a vegetative state remaining for longer than one month after acute traumatic or non-traumatic brain damage (The Multi-Society Task Force on Persistent Vegetative State 1994). It does not imply irreversibility, because it is a diagnostic, not a prognostic term. On the other hand, permanent vegetative state is irreversible (Jennet and Plum 1972, Medical Consultants on the Diagnosis of Death 1981, Jennet 2002).

However, there is some debate about the use of the terms permanent and persistent in relation to the vegetative state. Specifically, permanent vegetative state should be diagnosed only when there can be a high degree of certainty of irreversibility (Bernat 1992).

In essence, patients in a vegetative state are awake but, as far as can be determined, they are unaware of themselves or their environment (Jennett and Plum 1972, Jennett 2002). They typically lie with their eyes open while awake and closed while asleep, breathe spontaneously, have preserved autonomic function, and intact limb tendon and cranial nerve-innervated reflexes. They can blink and show eye and facial movements (expressions). Despite eye opening, these patients have no voluntary movements and there is often evidence for sleep/wake cycles with either complete or partial preservation of brainstem functions. It is particularly important to assess whether any movements made by a patient thought to be in the vegetative state are reflex or under voluntary control. In particular, clinicians should carefully look for signs of conscious behaviour in younger children presumed to be vegetative because of severe congenital brain damage (Ashwal et al. 1992, Ashwal 2004,

Shewmon et al. 1999). Quite interstingly, the same clinical picture may be seen as the result of the progression of degenerative neurological disorders affecting the cerebral cortex, including dementias (see chapter 6). The pathological basis of the persistent vegetative state is usually a widespread cortical damage resulting from such causes as cerebral hypoxia or widespread subcortical damage resulting from severe head injury.

In the 1990s two expert task forces (the Multisociety Task Force on Persistent Vegetative State in US and the Royal College of Physicians Working Group in UK) produced a series of clinical criteria for the definition of vegetative state (Multi-Society Task Force on PVS 1994, Royal College of Physicians Working Group 1996, Bauby 1997). There should be no evidence of awareness of self or environment at any time. There should be no volitional response to visual auditory, tactile or noxious stimuli. There should be no evidence of language comprehension or expression (Childs et al. 1993). There should be presence of cycles of eye closure and eye opening which may simulate sleep and wakening (Ostrum 1994). There should be sufficiently preserved hypothalamic and brainstem function to ensure the maintenance of respiration and circulation. The task forces acknowledged the biological limitations to knowing categorically that patients with vegetative state lack all awareness or capacity for suffering or experience because one person can not directly experience the conscious life of another (Multi-Society Task Force on PVS 1994). We can only interact with other people and make a reasoned judgment about their cognitive life on the basis of the quality of their responses to our stimuli. Therefore, it is possible that we incorrectly deny the presence of their conscious life when it exists simply because we cannot measure it (Mc Quillen 1991). Despite this limitation, there are compelling reasons to conclude that patients in vegetative state utterly lack sentience based on recent neuroimaging data (see paragraph 6).

4.3.4. Minimally Conscious State

Both coma and vegetative state are characterized by the complete absence of behavioral signs of self and environmental awareness. Vegetative state can be readily distinguished from coma by observing for spontaneous or elicited eye-opening, which signals that the reticular system is again active, generating a wakeful, yet unaware, state (Jennett and Plum 1972). Vegetative state is also distinguished from coma by the presence of the so-called "vegetative" functions of the body, namely respiration, heart rate and thermal regulation. The course of recovery from vegetative state is typically slow, with a gradual and subtle transition from unconsciousness to consciousness. Motor response to verbal command and discernible communication represent the clearest signs of reemerging consciousness, but these behaviors can occur inconsistently during the early stages of recovery, and are often difficult to differentiate from random movements (Giacino and Zasler 2005). Moreover, some patients fail to progress beyond this level of responsiveness and remain permanently incapable of consistently producing sentient behavior. These patients occupy an intermediate point along a continuum of consciousness that includes those in vegetative state on one pole, and those who consistently exhibit meaningful behavioural responses on the other. This intermediate subgroup of patients was indiscriminately lumped together with patients in vegetative state and coma, until the Aspen Neurobehavioral Conference expert panel formulated consensus-based diagnostic criteria for such patients whose clinical syndrome they termed the minimally conscious state (Giacino et al. 2002). They emphasised the qualitative difference between patients in minimally conscious state and vegetative state: although patients in both conditions are poorly responsive, those in a minimally conscious state show unequivocal - if intermittent and limited - evidence of awareness of themselves and their environment. (Giacino et al. 1997).

A key element of this new diagnostic category is the requirement that the behavior(s) of interest have to be viewed as unequivocally "meaningful" by the examiner, in other words they must represent a clear-cut behavioural sign of consciousness. From this perspective, minimally conscious state is defined as a condition of severely altered consciousness in which minimal but definite behavioural evidence of self or environmental awareness is demonstrated (Giacino et al. 2002). The diagnostic criteria for minimally conscious state rest largely on the integrity of the language and motor systems. To be minimally conscious, patients have to show limited but clear evidence of awareness of themself or their environment, by at least one of the following behaviours: following simple commands, gestural or verbal yes/no response (regardless of accuracy), intelligible speech, movements or affective behaviors that occur in contingent relation to relevant environmental stimuli and are not attributable to reflexive activity. Examples of contingent behavioural responses include episodes of crying, smiling, laughing, or vocalizations in response to the linguistic or visual content of emotional stimuli; reaching, touching or holding objects that demonstrate a clear relationship between object location and direction of reach; pursuit eye movement or sustained fixation that occurs in direct response to moving or salient stimuli. The behavior of interest must be reproducible during the examination and must be representative of cognitive processing. Emergence from the minimally conscious state is defined by the ability to communicate or use objects functionally (Giacino et al. 2002). Further improvement is more likely than in patients in a vegetative state (Giacino et al. 1997), although some people remain in a minimally conscious state permanently.

It has to be mentioned that the usefulness of creating a new diagnostic category for these disabled patients has been questioned. First, although patients in a minimally conscious state had markedly impaired responsiveness but demonstrable awareness, it did not necessarily follow that their consciousness was minimal, as implied by the name of their diagnosis. A more accurate term for them is "minimally responsive state" (Bernat 2002) as used in earlier reports and classification schemes (Whyte et al. 2005, Wilson et al. 2002). Second, disturbances of higher cognitive function, such as aphasia and apraxia, may confound assessment of clinical criteria and should be considered before establishing the diagnosis of minimally conscious state. Finally, some critics simply remain skeptical regarding the scientific justification for delineating a new and vaguely defined diagnostic category within the continuum of severely brain-injured patients (Shewmon et al. 2002).

4.3.5. Locked-in Syndrome

The term locked-in syndrome was first introduced by Plum and Posner (1983) to describe the clinical picture of total paralysis (quadriplegia) and inability to speak (anarthria) resulting from the disruption of the brainstem's corticospinal and corticobulbar descending pathways, respectively. Plum and Posner (1983) described the locked-in syndrome as "a state in which selective supranuclear motor de-efferentation produces paralysis of all four limbs and the last cranial nerves without interfering with consciousness. The voluntary motor paralysis prevents the subjects from communicating by word or body movement. Usually, but not always, the anatomy of the responsible lesion in the brainstem is such that locked-in patients are left with the capacity to use vertical eye movements and blinking to communicate their awareness of internal and external stimuli." Consequently, eye or eyelid movements (e.g. blinking of the upper eyelid to signal yes/no responses) are the main method of conscious experience communication (American Congress of Rehabilitation Medicine 1995).

Bauer et al. (1979) subdivided the syndrome on the basis of the extent of motor impairment: (a) classical locked-in syndrome is characterized by complete immobility except for vertical eye movements or blinking; (b) incomplete locked-in syndrome permits some voluntary motion; (c) total locked-in syndrome consists of total immobility (including all eye movements) combined with preserved consciousness. More recently, the American Congress of Rehabilitation Medicine (1995) defined locked-in syndrome by the following criteria: (i) presence of sustained eye opening; (ii) preserved basic cognitive abilities; (iii) aphonia or severe hypophonia; (iv) quadriplegia or quadriparesis; (v) a primary mode of communication that uses vertical or lateral eye movement or blinking of the upper eyelid.

The neuropathological basis for this condition is usually a bilateral lesion of the ventral pons and efferent motor tracks (e.g., Plum and Posner 1983, Patterson and Grabois 1986). In rarer instances, it can be the result of a mesencephalic lesion (e.g., Chia 1991; Meienberg et al. 1979, Bauer et al. 1979). The most common etiology of locked-in syndrome is vascular pathology, namely basilar artery occlusion. A similar clinical picture may sometimes be seen in patients with pontine tumours, pontine haemorrhage, central pontine myelinolysis, traumatic brain injury or brainstem encephalitis (Britt et al. 1977, Landrieu et al. 1984, Keane, 1986, Rae-Grant et al. 1989; Fitzgerald et al. 1997; Golubovic et al. 2004). In all cases recovery is exceptional (Plum and Posner 1983).

4.4. IMITATORS OF COMA

Stupor

Stupor is a state in which the patient, although not conscious, exhibits little or no spontaneous activity. In this state the individual appears to be asleep and yet, when vigorously stimulated, may become alert as manifest by eye opening and ocular movements. Other motor activities are limited and there is usually no speech. Although a proportion of patients in stupor have diffuse organic cerebral dysfunction, a variety of psychiatric disorders produce an identical clinical picture (Andrews et al. 1996, Childs et al. 1993). It may be difficult to differentiate stupor resulting from organic cerebral dysfunction from those with catatonic schizophrenia or severe depression.

Confusion

Confusion can be defined as a clouding of consciousness, characterised by impaired capacity to think clearly and with customary repetition, and to perceive, respond to and remember current stimuli; it is often associated with disorientation. It implies a generalized disturbance of brain function, especially of the cerebral cortex.

Delirium

Delirium is a transient state of agitated confusion, associated with motor restlessness, transient hallucinations, disorientation and possibly delusions. It can be caused by metabolic imbalances and is commonly observed in patients suffering from chronic alcoholism.

Akinetic Mutism

Akinetic mutism was first described by Cairns and colleagues (1941) in patients with damage to the bilateral orbitofrontal lobes. The clinical picture is characterised by immobility and eye closure with little or no vocalisation, whilst sleep/ wake cycles can be seen, as indicated by eye opening. Clinical and pathological evidence indicates that akinetic mutism can arise as a result of lesions of the bilateral cingulate gyrus that interfere with reticular cortical/integration (Devinsky et al. 1995, Mega and Cohenour 1997). This syndrome is not clearly differentiated from the early stages of the vegetative state.

Catatonia

The catatonic state is usually associated with psychiatric illness (affective or psychotic disorders) but may also occur in metabolic and drug-induced disorders. Despite being conscious, patients do not move spontaneously and seem unresponsive to their surroundings. Neurological examination is normal, but passive limb movements are met with a "waxy flexibility". It is often difficult to distinguish catatonia from organic disease, particularly in lethargic unresponsive individuals.

Psychogenic Coma

In psychogenic coma, subjects keep the eyelids firmly shut and are resistant to opening. Motor tone is normal or inconsistent and limb reflexes retained. Several physical signs based on reflex self protection have been used in the diagnosis of this syndrome although their validity has not been formally assessed.

4.5. THE ASSESSMENT OF THE UNRESPONSIVE PATIENT

The assessment of consciousness necessarily relies on the responses that a patient might give, and the actions that he might undertake, either spontaneously or as a response. Patients with profound impairment of consciousness are commonly assessed using specific tools, such as the Glasgow coma scale. This scale is probably the best method of assessing the level of consciousness, and has three components: eye, verbal and motor response to external stimuli (Table 4.1).

Teasdale and Jennett (1974) originally developed this scale for the clinical assessment of post-traumatic unconsciousness. It was devised as a formal scheme to overcome the ambiguities that arose when information about comatose patients was shared between specialists and carers.

Table 4.1. The Glasgow Coma Scale

Eye opening	Motor response	Verbal response
1- Absent	1- Absent	1- Absent
2- To pain	2- Abnormal extension	2- Incomprehensible
3- To verbal stimuli	3- Abnormal flexion	3- Comprehensible
4- Spontaneous	4- Weak flexion	4- Confused
	5- Localization	5- Fully orientated
	6- Obeys command	

The observation of spontaneous eye opening "indicates that the arousal mechanisms of the brainstem are active" Teasdale and Jennett (1974). However, recovered arousal does not imply the recovery of awareness. For instance, patients in a vegetative state have awakened from their coma but remain unaware of their environment and self. Most comatose patients who survive will eventually open their eyes, regardless of the severity of their cerebral damage (Jennett 1972). It has been reported that less than 4% of brain-damaged patients never open their eyes before they die (Bricolo et al. 1980). The eye opening in response to speech tests the reaction "to any verbal approach, whether spoken or shouted,not necessarily the command to open the eyes" (Teasdale and Jennett, 1974).

The presence of verbal responses indicates the restoration of a sufficient degree of interaction with the environment. A fully oriented conversation requires awareness of both the self and the environment. Confused speech is recorded when the patient is able to produce sentences but can not answer questions about orientation. When the patient presents intelligible articulations as isolated words pronounced in a random way, this is scored as inappropriate speech. Incomprehensible sounds refer to unrecognisable moaning or groaning: these rudimental vocalizations do not necessitate awareness and are thought to depend upon subcortical functioning.

The motor response assesses whether the patient obeys simple commands. For example, a non-specific sound stimulus may induce a reflex contraction of the fingers. Stereotyped flexion responses are the most common and enduring motor reactions observed in severely brain-injured patients (Born 1998). Abnormal flexion and extensor posturing often co-exist (Bricolo et al. 1977).

A significant limitation of the Glasgow Coma Scale is its failure to incorporate brainstem reflexes. A number of investigators have denied that spontaneous eye opening is sufficiently indicative of brainstem arousal systems activity and have proposed coma scales that include proper brainstem responses (Segatore and Way 1992). The Glasgow Liege Scale was developed in 1982 in Liège and combines the Glasgow Scale with a quantified analysis of five brainstem reflexes: fronto-orbicular, vertical oculo-cephalic, pupillary, horizontal oculo-cephalic and oculo-cardiac (Born et al. 1982). The fronto-orbicular reflex is considered present when percussion of the glabella produces contraction of the orbicularis oculi muscle. The oculo-cephalic reflexes (doll's head) are scored as present when deviation of at least one eye can be induced by vertical and horizontal neck movements, or by irrigation of the external auditory canal using iced water (i.e., oculo-vestibular reflex testing). The oculocardiac reflex is present when pressure on the eyeball causes the heart rate to slow down. The best response determines the brainstem reflex score. These reflexes disappear in descending order during rostral-caudal deterioration: the disappearance of the oculocardiac reflex coincides with brain death.

Table 4.2 summarizes and compares the behavioural characteristics of different unresponsive states. Table 4.3 shows how the two dimensions of consciousness (arousal = level; awareness = contents) vary in the unresponsive subject.

Table 4.2. Comparison of behavioural features of the main unresponsive states

Behavior	Locked-in	MCS	Vegetative state	Coma	Brain death
Respiratory function	Intact	Intact	Intact	Depressed/variable	Absent
Eye opening	Spontaneous	Spontaneous	Spontaneous	Absent	Absent
Spontaneous movement	Absent	Automatic/object manipulation	Reflex/patterned	Absent	Absent
Response to pain	Absent	Localization	Posturing/withdrawal	Posturing/Absent	Posturing/Absent
Visual response	Object recognition/pursuit	Object recognition/pursuit	Startle/pursuit (rare)	Absent	Absent
Affective response	Intact	Contingent	Random	Absent	Absent
Verbalization	Absent	Intelligible words	Random vocalization	Absent	Absent

MCS, minimally conscious state.
From Giacino 2005 (modified).

Table 4.3. Level and contents of consciousness in the unresponsive subject

Condition	Arousal/wakefulness (level of consciousness)	Awareness (contents of consciousness)
Brain death	↓	↓
Coma	↓	↓
Vegetative state	↑	↓
MCS	↑	↑↓
Locked-in	↑	↑

MCS, minimally conscious state.
From Laureys (2005), and Bernat (2006), modified.

4.6. THE BRAIN OF THE UNRESPONSIVE PATIENT

Studies of functional brain imaging with fMRI and PET have disclosed interesting findings that in some cases help discriminate vegetative state from coma, minimally conscious state, and other states of impaired consciousness (Laureys et al. 2004).

Brain Death

Brain death results from irreversible loss of brainstem function (Wijdicks 2001). Functional imaging studies with cerebral perfusion and metabolism tracers (Facco et al. 1998, Meyer 1996) typically show a "hollow skull phenomenon" in patients who are brain dead, thus confirming the absence of neuronal activity in the whole brain.

Coma

Coma can result from diffuse bihemispheric cortical or white-matter damage after neuronal or axonal injury, or from focal brainstem lesions that affect the pontomesencephalic region or paramedian thalami bilaterally. According to PET studies, grey matter metabolism is 50-70% of the normal range in comatose patients of traumatic or hypoxic origin (Schaafsma et al. 2003, Bergsneider et al. 2001). These metabolic rates are similar to levels of normal patients undergoing general anaesthesia (Alkire et al. 1997, Alkire et al. 1999). On the other hand, in patients who recover from a postanoxic coma there is a reduction of cerebral metabolic rates to 75% of the normal range (DeVolder et al. 1990).

Overall, these PET studies are not clinically useful, because they correlate poorly with the level of consciousness, as measured by the Glasgow Coma Scale (Hattori et al. 2003, Bergsneider et al. 2000), in patients studied within the first month after head trauma (Bergsneider et al. 2000). New generation PET scanning of comatose and noncomatose survivors of brain truma within 5 days of trauma has shown a correlation between the level of consciousness and the regional cerebral metabolism in the thalamus, brainstem, and cerebellar cortex (Hattori et al. 2003). The mechanisms underlying these changes in cerebral metabolism are not completely understood. At present, there is no established relation between cerebral metabolic rates of glucose or oxygen as measured by PET and patient outcome (Bergsneider et al. 2001).

Vegetative State

In a vegetative state the brainstem is mostly spared whereas both cerebral hemispheres are widely and severely damaged. Several studies of resting brain function in vegetative state by PET show a baseline decrease in cortical metabolism to 40–50% of the normal range of values (Levy et al. 1987, DeVolder et al. 1990, Tommasino et al. 1995, Rudolf et al. 1999, Boly et al. 2004). In "permanent" vegetative state (i.e. 12 months after a trauma or 3 months after nontraumatic brain damage), brain metabolism values drop to 30-40% of the normal range of values (Tommasino et al. 1995). The relative sparing of metabolism of the brainstem and allied structures maintains arousal and autonomic functions in these patients (Laureys et al. 2000). Polymodal associative cortices (posterior parietal areas and precuneus, bilateral prefrontal regions, Broca's area, and parietotemporal area) (Laureys et al. 1999) are particularly affected (Laureys et al. 2004) as is their connectivity (Laureys et al. 2002). These regions are important in various functions that are necessary for consciousness, such as attention, memory, and language (Baars et al. 2003). It is not known whether the observed metabolic impairment in this large cortical network reflects an irreversible structural neuronal loss, (Rudolf et al. 2000) or functional and potentially reversible damage. However, in rare cases where patients in a vegetative state recover awareness of self and environment, PET shows a concomitant improvement in both cortical metabolism (Rudolf et al. 1999) and connectivity (Laureys et al. 2000) in these same cortical regions (Laureys et al. 1999). The resumption of functional connectivity between these associative cortices (Laureys et al. 1999) and between some of these and the intralaminar thalamic nuclei parallels the restoration of their functional integrity (Laureys et al. 2000). These data suggest that the observed baseline reduction in resting cerebral metabolism represents a combination of potentially reversible neuronal metabolic dysfunction and irreversible neuronal death (Laureys et al. 2000).

Minimally Conscious State

There are very few functional imaging studies of patients in this newly defined condition. Preliminary data show that overall cerebral metabolism is decreased to values slightly higher than those observed in the vegetative state. In a PET study, Laureys et al. (2000) exposed a patient in minimally conscious state to no sound, frequency-modulated noise, infant cries and the patient's own voice. Although global metabolism was significantly reduced relative to controls, activation spread to heteromodal association cortices following presentation of the infant cries and the patient's name. Functionally connectivity analyses performed in other PET paradigms have also shown significantly greater activation of medial parietal, posterior cingulate, and secondary frontal and temporal cortices in minimally conscious state patients, relative to those in vegetative state (Laureys et al. 2003). The lack of activity in these regions in vegetative state has been correlated with the presumed absence of cognitive processing in this condition. In particular, the medial parietal cortex (precuneus) and adjacent posterior cingulate cortex seem to be the crucial brain regions that differentiate patients in minimally conscious state from those in vegetative state (Laureys et al. 2003). Interestingly, these richly connected (Vogt et al. 1995) multimodal posteromedial associative areas are among the most active brain regions in conscious waking (Teasdale and Jennett 1974, Andreasen et al. 1995, Maquet et al. 1997, Gusnard and Raichle 2001) and are among the least active regions in altered states of consciousness. It has been suggested that they may play a key role in the neural network subserving general awareness (Cavanna and Trimble 2006).

Locked-in Syndrome

Classically, structural brain imaging (MRI) of locked-in patients shows isolated lesions (bilateral infarction, hemorrhage, or tumor) of the ventral portion of the basis pontis or midbrain (e.g. Leon-Carrion et al. 2002). While neurophysiological tests (EEG and evoked potentials) do not seem to reliably distinguish the locked-in syndrome from the vegetative state (Gutling et al. 1996), PET scanning has shown higher metabolic levels in the brains of patients in a locked-in syndrome compared to those in a vegetative state (Levy et al. 1987). Preliminary PET studies by Laureys et al. (2003) indicate that no supra-tentorial cortical area show significantly lower metabolism in locked-in syndrome patients when compared to healthy subjects (Laureys et al. 2003). The absence of metabolic signs of reduced activity in any cortical area emphasizes the fact that locked-in syndrome patients suffer from a pure motor de-efferentation and recover an entirely intact intellectual capacity. Conversely, locked-in patients displayed increased regional activity within the amigdalar nuclei. Several PET studies in normal volunteers have shown amygdalar activation in relation to negative emotions such as fear and anxiety (e.g. Calder et al. 2001). It is difficult to make judgments about patient's thoughts and feelings when they awake from their coma speechless and in a motionless shell. However, in the absence of decreased neural activity in any cortical region, it has been assumed that the increased amigdalar activity relates to the terrifying situation of an intact self-awareness in a sensitive being, experiencing frustration, stress and anguish, locked in an immobile body.

4.7. DRUG-INDUCED ANESTHESIA: INDUCTION AND RECOVERY

It has been claimed that anesthesiologists are in a unique situation, as they strive to understand the complex nature of anesthesia, but the targets for the drugs they use are still poorly defined (Fiset 2003). Based on a huge amount of empirical knowledge and advanced clinical research, they are now able to modulate very precisely the state of consciousness of their patients, but can not provide a comprehensive explanation of the brain processes involved. In daily practice anesthesiologists usually refer to consciousness and awareness synonymously, being interested in the practical aspects of patient care and concerned about the possibility that a patient might be aware during surgical procedures. On the other hand, by investigating how anesthetic drugs affect neural targets, anesthesia researchers have refined the understanding of how central nervous system networks support consciousness. Anesthetic drugs are used not only to render patients unconscious, but also to induce a whole range of sedative states in a precise and controlled fashion. It is possible to induce, in any individual, a controlled change of conscious state along a wide range of behavioural states.

Anesthetic drugs can produce predictable, reversible changes in the level of consciousness that range from light sedation to complete unresponsiveness. Given a sufficient dose of anesthesia, a number of different anesthetics are able to stop the brain's spontaneous electrical activity, as measured by flat or isoelectric electroencephalographic (EEG) recordings (Drummond and Patel 2000). It is assumed that when the brain is in such a state, then consciousness is completely lost and it becomes impossible for a person under anesthesia to perceive anything. Anesthetic drugs can be titrated to achieve specific behavioural endpoints and precise alterations in level of consciousness. The administration of anesthetic drugs is based on a solid scientific foundation and relates to the fundamental concept of concentration-effect relationships. The concentration needed to achieve a given behavioural change has been the subject of numerous studies and is well known for several anesthetic drugs, including inhalation anesthetics, benzodiazepines, propofol, barbiturates, opioids and ketamine. Research has not only been conducted during the administration of single drugs, but also using drug combinations to determine their synergistic effects (Vuyk et al. 1997, Kazama et al. 1998).

Moreover, the influence weight (Egan et al. 1998), gender, and age (Minto et al. 1997, Dyck and Shafer 1992), is now routinely determined and translated into standard recommendations for dosing. The net result is a better and safer context for the administration of anesthesia to patients; moreover this knowledge, when applied to research on anesthetic drug action and consciousness, represents the basis for our understanding of changes occurring in the central nervous system. Sophisticated tools for administration of drugs are currently available. For volatile anesthetics, drugs dose can be controlled by measuring the expired concentration, which is an approximation of plasma drug concentration. For intravenous agents, direct plasma concentration measurement is not yet possible, but the availability of computer-controlled infusion pumps allows the researcher to obtain target plasma drug concentrations with striking precision (Vuyk et al. 1995, Swinhoe et al. 1998).

These devices use population pharmacokinetics to determine the infusion rate needed to immediately reach and maintain a target plasma concentration. (Shafer and Gregg 1992, Varvel et al. 1992, Vuyk et al. 1995).

In summary, the study of anesthetic drug effect on the central nervous system is based on the knowledge of concentration-effect relationships and on the availability of tools that allow for obtaining stable plasma concentrations. Consciousness represents a dependent variable that can be directly manipulated using the power of anesthetic drugs (Alkire et al. 1998). In the following section, a few examples will be given to illustrate how we can use anesthetic drugs to induce controlled modulation of conscious functions in order to uncover their neural correlates.

4.8. FUNCTIONAL IMAGING OF GENERAL ANESTHESIA

Brain imaging is the most powerful tool for identifying central nervous system sites affected by anesthetic drugs. Recent advances in the development of target-specific anesthetic agents coupled with advances in molecular neurobiology and neuroimaging techniques permit a sophisticated approach to studying how anesthetic drugs act on the central nervous system. This approach is based on the premise that anesthetics induce localized changes in neuronal function, which in turn can be assessed by measuring changes in blood flow.

Thus, when anesthetic manipulation is coupled with recent advances in brain imaging techniques, a powerful method emerges that can provide answers to some fundamental questions about the anatomy of consciousness. Recent functional neuroimaging studies have provided a basic understanding of how anesthesia affects cerebral blood flow (CBF) and cerebral metabolic rate (CMR) in humans (Drummond and Patel 2000). Overall, most anesthetic agents decrease global cerebral metabolism in a dose-dependent fashion with variable effects on global cerebral blood flow (Heinke and Schwarzbauer 2002). Furthermore, the regional effects of several anesthetic agents have been studied with neuroimaging in humans at doses near to those required to produce complete unconsciousness. In experimental settings, the "unconscious" endpoint is the dose of anesthetic at which it causes a subject to be unable to respond to verbal or physical stimulation. This end-point occurs at low anesthetic dose relative to the dose needed for an operation, which would cause an isoelectric EEG. It has been hypothesized that the loss of consciousness induced by general anesthetic agents may result, at least in part, from a disruption of functional interactions within distributed neural networks involving the thalamus and the cerebral cortex, i.e. the structures involved in the control of the level of consciousness (Sugiyama et al. 1992; Angel 1993, Ries and Puil 1999, Alkire et al. 2000).

For the anesthetic end-point of loss of consciousness in humans, a more recent case has been made for a common effect of most agents on thalamic metabolism and thalamocortical-corticothalamic connectivity (AIkire et al. 2000, White and Alkire, 2003). This observation led to the development of the "thalamic consciousness switch" hypothesis of anesthetic-induced unconsciousness (Alkire et al. 2000). *In vivo* electrophysiological work in animals has provided compelling evidence that anesthetic have an ability to affect thalamocortical signalling (Angel 1993, Steriade 2001). It has been shown that anesthetic agents compromise the natural firing patterns of thalamic network neurons (i.e. thalamocortical, corticothalamic, and reticulothalamic cells) by hyperpolarizing their resting membrane potentials (Nicoll and Madison 1982, Berg-Johnsen and Langmoen 1987, Steriade et al. 2001). This in turn blocks synaptic transmission of sensory information through the thalamus and diminishes the high frequency rhythms that characterize the spontaneous activity associated with the awake state and dreaming experiences (Angel 1991, Llinas and Pare 1991, Lytton and Sejnowski 1991, Buzsaki and Chrobak 1995, Steriade 2000). It has been hypothesized that anesthetics may cause unconsciousness in the human brain because they induce a hyperpolarization blockade that involves a sufficient proportion of the thalamocortical cells and networks that are required for the maintenance of conscious awareness (Sugiyama et al. 1992, Ries and Puil 1999, Alkire et al. 2000).

Sleep and anesthesia share a number of physiological and behavioural traits (Lydic and Biebuyck 1994) in particular, the fact that they both result in a loss of consciousness suggests that they may share some common mechanistic features. When the hypothesis of the "thalamic consciousness switch" was originally developed in relation to human neuroimaging (Alkire et al. 2000), it took into account regional cerebral blood flow effects on the thalamus that were observed in humans as a site of a common overlapping effect between hypnotic drugs - the benzodiazepines lorazepam (Volkow et al. 1995) and midazolam (Veselis et al. 1997) - and anesthetic agents - propofol (Fiset et al. 1999), isoflorane and halothane (Alkire et al. 2000). Further additional study has remained consistent with the thalamic overlap effect and has shown replications of propofol's thalamic effects (Kaisti et al. 2003; Veselis et al. 2004), along with an overlapping thalamic effect for the additional inhalational anesthetic agent sevoflurane (Kaisti et al. 2002).

Overall, despite the often dramatic technical differences between studies, what emerges is that when consciousness goes away with any number of different anesthetics, a relative decrease in thalamic activity occurs. This effect implies that there is a minimal amount of regional thalamic activity that may be necessary to maintain consciousness, and the thalamus or thalamocortical networks, therefore, emerge as potentially amportant components of the neural correlates of general awareness. The centralized placement of the thalamus within the brain and its unique direct access to all incoming sensory information, along with its access to cortical feedback, places this structure at the center of interest as a brain region that might play a central role in the mechanisms of consciousness and attention (Newman 1997a,b).

In fact, impairments of consciousness are known to occur with even relatively small bilateral lesions of the thalamus (see Figure 4.1), especially those involving the intralaminar nuclei (see e.g. Bogen 1997). The intralaminar nuclei and the thalamic reticular nucleus are considered an extension of the brainstem reticular activating system (Newman 1997a,b) and anesthetic effects on the brainstem reticular activating system have long been associated with anesthetic effects on consciousness (Moruzzi and Magoun 1949).

The second most consistent anesthetic-related regional overlap effect involves the medial parietal cortical areas. In a classical PET study, Fiset et al. (1999) investigated changes in rCBF during a general anaesthetic infusion, set to produce a gradual transition from the awake state to unconsciousness. In addition to a generalized decrease in global cerebral blood flow, propofol-induced anaesthesia was characterised by marked regional flow decrements in the precuneus, the posterior cingulate, the cuneus, the medial thalamus and frontal cortical regions. These findings support the hypothesis that anaesthetics induce behavioural changes via an effect on specific neuronal networks, that are implicated in the regulation of arousal and performance of associative conscious functions. These richly interconnected multimodal associative areas located in the medial surface of the parietal cortex are a key region of the neural network subserving awareness and conscious experience. The central nervous system areas primarily affected by propofol were those typically involved in the maintenance of the conscious state, but also those that are active at the resting state (Gusnard and Raichle 2001).

They compared these results with those from other studies in which consciousness had been lost during sleep or coma. Some areas common to all forms of altered consciousness were deactivated, like the precuneus, posterior cingulate and cuneus. They hypothesized that these areas are part of a network that is responsible for the existence of a baseline resting state of the brain, a state that allows us to be awake, and ready to process incoming information. This concept, also referred to as the "default mode of brain function"(Binder et al. 1999, Mazoyer et al. 2001) is the subject of a growing interest in neuroscience related to consciousness (Greicius et al. 2003).

A variety of neurotransmitters and modulators appear to be affected by anesthetic drugs, however most studies have focused on the role of acetylcholine. Compelling evidence from *in vivo* animal sleep studies suggests that altered central cholinergic drive can mediate changes in endogenous states of consciousness (Steriade 1990). Both *in vitro* and *in vivo* studies demonstrate that a variety of anesthetic drugs interfere with cholinergic transmission (Lydic and Baghdoyan 1997). In addition, in both human and animal experiments, the anesthetic-induced depression of the central nervous system is augmented by cholinergic (muscarinic) antagonists (Ali-Melkkila et al. 1993).

This view is supported by a number of anecdotal reports in which physostigmine, an acetylcholinesterase (AChe) inhibitor that crosses the blood-brain barrier, decreased the time to awaken from anesthesia, and modulated or simply reversed the effect of anesthetic drugs on consciousness. These results suggest that the muscarinic system, which plays an important role in the maintenance of the conscious state (Durieux 1996) is affected by the administration of anesthetic drugs. Converging evidence points towards the thalamus, thalamocortical, and corticocortical interactions as being critically involved with mediating not only anesthetic induced unconsciousness, but also with mediating other forms of altered states of consciousness. However, the study of the effects of anesthetics on consciousness is at its very beginning. While these pioneering PET studies have great merit as panoramic windows of neural network correlates of consciousness, wider ranges of theory and empirical evidence need to be brought into the formulation of truly comprehensive theories of consciousness and anesthesia.

4.9. REFERENCES

Alkire MT, Haier RJ, Fallon JH. Toward a unified theory of narcosis: brain imaging evidence for a thalamocortical switch as the neurophysiologic basis of anaesthetic-induced unconsciousness. *Conscious Cogn.* 2000;9:370-386.

Ali-Melkkila T, Kanto J, Lisalo E. Pharmacokinects and related pharmacodynamics of anticholinergic drugs. *Acta Anaesthesiol Scand. 1993;*37:633-642.

Alkire MT, Haier RJ, Shah NK, Anderson CT. Positron emission tomography study of regional cerebral metabolism in humans during isofl urane anesthesia. *Anesthesiology.*1997;86:549-57.

Alkire MT, Pomfrett CJ, Haier RJ, Gianzero MV, Chan CM, Jacobsen BP, Fallon JH. Functional brain imaging during anesthesia in humans: effects of halothane on global and regional glucose metabolism. *Anesthesiology.*1999;90:701-09.

American Congress of Rehabilitation Medicine. Recommendations for use of uniform nomenclature pertinent to patients with severe alterations of consciousness. *Arch Phys Med Rehabil.* 1995;76:205–9.

Andreasen NC, O'Leary DS, Cizadlo T, Amdt S, Rezai K, Watkins GL, Ponto LL, Hichwa RD. Remembering the past: two facets of episodic memory explored with positron emission tomography. *Am J Psychiatry.* 1995;152:1576–85.

Andrews K, Murphy L, Munday R, Littlewood C. Misdiagnosis of the vegetative state: retrospective study in a rehabilitation unit. *Br Med J.* 1996;313:13-16.

Angel A. Adventures in anaesthesia. *Exp Physiol.* 1991;76:1-38.

Angel A. Central neuronal pathways and the process of anaesthesia. *Br J Anaesth.* 2003;71:148-163.

Ashwal S, Bale JF, Coulter DL, Eiben R, Garg BP, Hill A, Myer EC, Nordgren RE, Shewmon DA, Sunder TR. The persistent vegetative state in children: report of the Child Neurology Society Ethics Committee. *Ann Neurol.* 1992;32:570–76.

Ashwal S. Pediatric vegetative state: epidemiological and clinical issues. *NeuroRehabilitation.* 2004;19:349–60.

Baars BJ, Ramsoy T, Laureys S. Brain, conscious experience and the observing self. *Trends Neurosci.* 2003;26:671–75.

Bauby JD. *The diving bell and the butterfly.* Knopf, New York 1997.

Bauer G, Gerstenbrand F, Rumpl E. Varieties of the locked-in syndrome. *J Neurol.* 1979;221:77-91.

Berg-Johnsen J, Langmoen IA. Isoflurane hyperpolarizes neurones in rat and human cerebral cortex. *Acta Physiol Scand.* 1987;130:679-685.

Bergsneider M, Hovda DA, Lee SM, Kelly DF, Mc Arthur D, Phelps ME. Dissociation of cerebral glucose metabolism and level of consciousness during the period of metabolic depression following human traumatic brain injury. *J Neurotrauma.* 2000;17:389-401.

Bergsneider M, Hovda DA, McArthur DL, Etchepare M, Huang SC, Sehati N, Satz P, Phelps ME, Becker DP. Metabolic recovery following human traumatic brain injury based on FDG-PET: time course and relationship to neurological disability. *J Head Trauma Rehabil.* 2001;16:135-48.

Bernat JL. *Ethical issues in neurology,* 2nd edn. Butterworth-Heinemann, Boston 2002:283–305.

Bernat JL. The boundaries of the persistent vegetative state. *J Clin Ethics.* 1992;3:176–80.

Binder JR, Frost JA, Hammeke TA, Bellgowan PSF, Rao SM, Cox RW. Conceptual processing during the conscious resting state: a functional MRI study. *J Cogn Neurosci.* 1999;11:80-93.

Bogen J. Some neurophysiologic aspects of consciousness. *Semin Neurol.* 1997;17:95-103.

Boly M, Faymonville M-E, Peigneux P. Auditory processing in severely brain-injured patients: differences between the minimally conscious state and the persistent vegetative state. *Arch Neurol.* 2004;61:233–38.

Born JD, Hans P, Dexters G, Kalangu K, Lenelle J, Milbouw G, Stevenaert A. Practical assessment of brain dysfunction in severe head trauma. *Neurochirurgie,*1982;28:1-7.

Born. The Glasgow-Liège scale. Prognostic value and evaluation of motor response and brain stem reflexes after severe head injury. *Acta Neurochir.* 1998;95:49-52.

Borthwick CJ, Crossley R. Permanent vegetative state: usefulness and limits of a prognostic definition. *NeuroRehabilitation.* 2004;19:381–89.

Bricolo A, Turazzi S, Feriotti G. Prolonged posttraumatic unconsciousness:therapeutic assets and liabilitie. *J Neurosurg.* 1980;52:625-34.

Bricolo A, Turazzi S, Alexandre A, Rizzato N. Decerebrate rigidity in acute head injury. *J Neurosurg.* 1977;47:680-89.

Britt RH, Herrick MK, Hamilton RD. Traumatic locked-in syndrome. *Ann Neurol.* 1977;1:590-592.

Buzsaki G, Chrobak JJ. Temporal structure in spatially organized neuronal ensembles:a role for interneuronal networks. *Curr Opin Neurobiol.* 1995;5:504-510.

Cairns H, Oldfield RC, Pennybacker JB, Whitteridge D. Akinetic mutism with epidermoid cyst of the third ventricle (with a report on associated disturbance of brain potentials). *Brain.* 1941;64:273–90.

Chia S. Locked-in syndrome with bilateral ventral midbrain infarcts. *Neurology.* 1991;41:445-446.

Childs NL, Mercer WN, Childs HW. Accuracy of diagnosis of persistent vegetative state. *Neurology.* 1993;43:1465–67.

Devinsky O, Morrell MJ, Vogt BA. Contributions of anterior cingulate gyrus to behavior. *Brain.* 1995;118:273–90.

DeVolder AG, Goffinet AM, Bol A, Michel C, de Barsy T, Laterre C. Brain glucose metabolism in postanoxic syndrome: positron emission tomographic study. *Arch Neurol.* 1990;47:197-204.

Drummond P, Patel G. *Cerebral blood flow and metabolism.* In: Miller RD ed. Anesthesia. Churchill Livingstone, New York 2000. pp. 1203-1256.

Durieux ME. Muscarinic signaling in the central nervous system. Recent developments and anesthetic implications. *Anesthesiology.* 1996;84:173-89.

Dyck JB, Shafer SL. Effects of age on propofol pharmacokinetics. *Semin Anesth.* 1992;11:2-4.

Egan TD, Huizinga B, Gupta S, Jaarsma RL, Sperry RJ, Yee JB, Muir KT. Remifentanil pharmacokinetics in obese versus lean patients. *Anesthesiology.* 1998;89:562–73.

Facco E, Zucchetta P, Munari M. 99mTc-HMPAO SPECT in the diagnosis of brain death. *Intensive Care Med.* 1998;24:911-17.

Fiset P, Paus T, Daloze T, Plourde G, Meuret P, Bonhomme V. Brain mechanisms of propofol-induced loss of consciousness in humans: a positron emission tomographic study. *J Neurosci.* 1999;19:5506-13.

Fitzgerald JD, Mangione CM, Boscardin J, Kominski G, Hahn B, Ettner SL. Locked-in syndrome resulting from cervical spine gunshot wound. *J Trauma.* 1997;42:147-49.

Giacino JT and Zasler ND. Outcome after severe traumatic brain injury:Coma,the vegetative state,and the minimally responsive state. *J Head Trauma Rehabil.* 2005;10:40-56.

Giacino JT. Development of practice guidelines for the assessment and management of the vegetative and minimally conscious states. *J Head Trauma Rehabil.* 1997;12:79-89.

Giacino JT, Ashwal S, Childs N et al. The minimally conscious state: definition and diagnostic criteria. *Neurology.* 2002;58:349–53.

Gill-Thwaites H, Munday R. The Sensory Modality Assessment and Rehabilitation Technique (SMART): a valid and reliable assessment for vegetative and minimally conscious patients. *Brain Inj.* 2004;18:1255–69.

Golubovic V, Muhvic D, Golubovic S. Post traumatic locked-in syndrome with an unusual three day delay in the appearance. *Coll Anthropol.* 2004;28:923-26.

Greicius MD, Krasnow B, Reiss AL, Menon V. Functional connectivity in the resting brain: a network analysis of the default mode hypothesis. *Proc Natl Acad Sci.* 2003;100:253-8.

Gusnard DA, Raichle ME. Searching for a baseline:functional imaging and the resting human brain. *Nat Rev Neurosci.* 2001;2:685-94.

Gutling E, Isenmann S, Wichmann W. Electrophysiology in the locked-in-syndrome. *Neurology.* 1996;46:1092-101.

Hattori N, Huang SC, Wu HM, Yeh E, Glenn TC, Vespa PM, Mc Arthur D, Phelps ME, Hovda DA, Bergsneider M. Correlation of regional metabolic rates of glucose with Glasgow Coma Scale after traumatic brain injury. *J Nucl Med.* 2003;44:1709-16.

Heinke W, Schwarzbauer C. In vivo imaging of anaesthetic action in humans: approaches with positron emission tomography (PET) and functional magnetic resonance imaging (MRI). *Br J Anaesth.* 89:112-122.

Jennett B, Plum F. Persistent vegetative state after brain damage: a syndrome in search of a name. *Lancet.* 1972;1:734–37.

Jennett B. Prognosis after severe head injury. *Clin. Neurosurg.* 1979;19:200-207.

Jennett B. The vegetative state: medical facts,ethical and legal dilemmas. Cambridge University Press, Cambridge 2002.

Kaisti KK, Langsjo JW, Aalto S, Oikonen V, Sipila H, Teras M, Hinkka S, Metsahonkala L, Scheinin H. Effects of sevoflurane, propofol, and adjunct nitrous oxide on regional cerebral blood flow, oxygen consumption, and blood volume in humans. *Anaesthesiology.* 2003;99:603-613.

Kaisti KK, Langsjo JW, Aalto S, Oikonen V, Sipila H, Teras M, Hinkka S, Metsahonkala L, Scheinin H. Effects of surgical levels of propofol and sevoflurane anesthesia on cerebral blood flow in healthy subjects studied with positron emission tomography. *Anaesthesiology.* 2002;96:1358-1370.

Kazama T, Ikeda K, Morita K. The pharmacodynamic interaction between propofol and fentanyl with respect to the suppression of somatic or hemodynamic responses to skin incision, peritoneum incision, and abdominal wall retraction. *Anesthesiology.* 1998;89:894-906.

Keane S. Locked-in syndrome after head and neck trauma. *Neurology. 1986;*36:80-82.

Landrieu P, Fromentin C, Tardieu M, Menget A, Laget P. Locked-in syndrome with a favourable outcome. *Eur J Pediatr.* 1984;142:144-145.

Laureys S. Differences in brain metabolism between patients in coma, vegetative state, minimally conscious state and locked-in syndrome. *Eur J Neurol. 2003* (suppl.1):224.

Laureys S, Antoine S, Boly M, Elincx S, Faymonville ME, Berre J, Sadzot B, Ferring M, De Tiege X, Hansen I, Lambermont B, Del Fiore G, Phillips C, Franck G, Lamy M, Maquet P. Brain function in the vegetative state. *Acta Neurol Belg.* 2002; 102:177–85.

Laureys S, Faymonville ME, Goldman S. *Impaired cerebral connectivity in vegetative state.* In:Gjedde A, Hansen SB, Knudsen GM, Paulson OB, eds. Physiological imaging of the brain with PET. Academic Press, San Diego 2000, 329–34.

Laureys S, Faymonville M-E, Luxen A, Lamy M, Franck G, Maquet P. Restoration of thalamocortical connectivity after recovery from persistent vegetative state. *Lancet.* 2000;355:1790–91.

Laureys S, Faymonville M-E, Moonen, Luxen A, Maquet P. PET scanning and neuronal loss in acute vegetative state. *Lancet* 2000;355:1825–26.

Laureys S, Goldman S, Phillips C. Impaired effective cortical connectivity in vegetative state: preliminary investigation using PET. *Neuroimage.* 1999;9:377–82.

Laureys S, Owen AM, Schiff ND. Brain function in coma, vegetative state, and related disorders. *Lancet Neurol.* 2004;3:537-46.

Laureys S. Functional neuroimaging in the vegetative state. *NeuroRehabilitation.* 2004;19:335–41.

Leon-Carrion J, van Eeckhout P, Dominguez-Morales Mdel R, Perez-Santamaria FJ. The locked-in syndrome:a syndrome looking for a theraphy. *Brain Inj.* 2002;16:571-582.

Levy DE, Bates D, Caronna JJ, Cartlidge NE, Knill-Jones RP, Lapinski RH, Singer BH, Shaw DA, Plum F. Prognosis in non traumatic coma. *Ann Intern Med* 1981;94:293-301.

Levy DE, Sidtis JJ, Rottenberg DA, Jarden JO, Strother SC, Dhawan V, Ginos JZ, Tramo MJ, Evans AC, Plum F. Differences in cerebral blood flow and glucose utilization in vegetative versus locked-in patients. *Ann Neurol.* 1987;22:673-82.

Lydic R, Baghdoyan HA. *Cholinergic contribution to the control of consciousness.* In: Yaksh TL ed. Anaesthesia: Biologic foundations. Lippincott Raven, Philadelphia 1997, pp.433-450.

Lydic R, Biebuyck JF. Sleep neurobiology: relevance for mechanistic studies of anaesthesia. *Br J Anaesth.* 1994;72:506–8.

Lytton WW, Sejnowski TJ. Simulations of cortical pyramidal neurons synchronized by inhibitory interneurons. *J Neurophysiol.* 1991;66:1059-1079.

Maquet P, Degueldre C, Delfiore G, Aerts J, Peters JM, Luxen A, Franck G. Functional neuroanatomy of human slow wave sleep. *J Neurosci.* 1997;17:2807-12.

Mazoyer B, Zago L, Mellet E, Bricogne S, Etard O. Cortical networks for working memory and executive functions sustain the conscious resting state in man. *Brain Res Bull.* 2001;54:287–98.

McQuillen MP. Can people who are unconscious or who are in the persistent vegetative state feel pain? *Issues Law Med.* 1991;6:373–83.

Medical Consultants on the Diagnosis of Death. Guidelines for the determination of death: report of the medical consultants on the diagnosis of death to the president's commission for the Study of Ethical Problems in Medicine and Biomedical and Behavioral Research. *J Am Med Assoc.* 1981;246:2184-6.

Mega MS, Cohenour RC. Akinetic mutism: disconnection of frontal-subcortical circuits. *Neuropsychiat Neuropsychol Behav Neurol.* 1997;10:254–59.

Meienberg O, Mumenthaler M, Karbowski K. Quadriparesis and nuclear oculomotor palsy with total bilateral ptosis mimicking coma: a mesencephalic "locked-in syndrome"? *Arch Neurol.* 1979;36:708-710.

Meyer MA. Evaluating brain death with positron emission tomography: case report on dynamic imaging of 18F-fluorodeoxyglucose activity after intravenous bolus injection. *J Neuroimaging.* 1996;6:117-19.

Minto CF, Schnider TW, Egan TD, Youngs E, Lemmens HJ, Gambus PL, Billard V, Hoke
    JF, Moore KH, Hermann DJ, Muir KT, Mandema JW, Shafer SL. Influence of age and
    gender on the pharmacokinetics and pharmacodynamics of remifentanil I. Model
    development. *Anesthesiology*. 1997;86:10–23.

Moruzzi M, Magoun H. Brain stem reticular formation and activation of the EEG.
    Electroencephal Clin Neurophysiol. 1949;1:455-473.

Newman LA. Llinas R, Pare. Of dreaming and wakefulness. *Neuroscience*. 1991;44:521-535.

Newman LA. Putting the puzzle together. Part I: towards a general theory of the neural
    correlates of consciousness. *J Consciousness Stud.* 2000a;4:46-66.

Newman LA. Putting the puzzle together. Part II: towards a general theory of the neural
    correlates of consciousness. *J Consciousness Stud.* 2000b;4:100-121.

Nicoll RA, Madison DV. General anesthetics hyperpolarize neurons in the vertebrate central
    nervous system. *Science*. 1982;217:1055-1057.

Ostrum AE. The 'locked-in' syndrome—comments from a survivor. *Brain Inj.* 1994;8:95-98.

Patterson JR, Grabois M. Locked-in syndrome:a rewiew of 139 cases. *Stroke.*1986;17:758-
    764.

Plum F, Posner JB. *The diagnosis of stupor and coma* (3rd edn). FA Davis, Philadelphia
    1983.

Rae-Grant AD, Lin F, Yaeger BA, Barbour P, Levitt LP, Castaldo JE, Lester MC. Post
    traumatic extracranial vertebral artery dissection with locked-in syndrome: a case with
    MRI documentation and unusually favourable outcome. *J Neurol Neurosurg Psychiatry*.
    1989;52:1191-93.

Ries CR, Puil E. Mechanism of anaesthesia revealed by shunting actions of isoflurane on
    thalamocortical neurons. *J Neurophysiol*. 1999;81:1795-1801.

Royal College of Physicians Working Group. The permanent vegetative state. *J R Coll
    Physicians Lond.* 1996;30:119–21.

Rudolf J, Ghaemi M, Haupt WF, Szelies B, Heiss WD. Cerebral glucose metabolism in acute
    and persistent vegetative state. *J Neurosurg Anesthesiol.* 1999;11:17–24.

Rudolf J, Sobesky J, Grond M, Heiss WD. Identification by positron emission tomography of
    comatose and vegetative state patients. *J Neurosurg Anesthesiol.* 1995;7:109-16.

Schaafsma A, de Jong BM, Bams JL, Haaxma-Reiche H, Pruim J, Zijlstra JG. Cerebral
    perfusion and metabolism in resuscitated patients with severe post-hypoxic
    encephalopathy. *J Neurol Sci.* 2003;210:23-30.

Shewmon DA, Holmes GL, Byrne PA. Consciousness in congenitally decorticate children:
    developmental vegetative state as self-fulfi lling prophecy. *Dev Med Child Neurol.* 1999;
    41:364-74.

Shewmon DA. The minimally conscious state: definition and diagnostic criteria. *Neurology.*
    2002; 58:506.

Steriade M, Timofeev I, Grenier F. Natural waking and sleep states:a view from inside
    neocortical neurons. *J Neurophysiol.* 2001;85:1969-1985.

Steriade M. Cholinergic control of thalamic function. *Archives Internationales de
    Physiologie et de Biochimie*. 1990;98:A11-A46.

Steriade M. Corticothalamic resonance, states of vigilance and mentation. *Neuroscience*.
    2000;101:243-276.

Steriade M. Impact of network activities on neuronal properties in corticothalamic systems. *J Neurophysiol.* 2001;86:1-39.

Sugiyama K, Muteki T, Shimoji K. Halothane-induced hyperpolarization and depression of postsynaptic potentials of guinea pig thalamic neurons in vitro. *Brain Res.* 2002;576:97-103.

Swinhoe CF, Peacock JE, Glen JB, Reilly CS. Evaluation of the predictive performance of a "Diprifusor" TCI system. *Anaesthesia.* 1998;53:61-7.

Teasdale G, Jennett B. Assessment of coma and impaired consciousness. *Lancet.* 1974;2:81-84.

The Multi-Society Task Force on Persistent Vegetative State. Medical aspects of the persistent neuronal loss in acute vegetative state. *Lancet.* 2000;355:155.

Tommasino C, Grana C, Lucignani G, Torri G, Fazio F. Regional cerebral metabolism of glucose in vegetative state. *N Engl J Med.* 1994;330:1499–508.

Veselis RA, Feshchenko VA, Reinsel RA, Dnistrian AM, Beattie B, Akhurst TJ. Thiopental and propofol affect different regions of the brain at similar pharmacologic effects. *Anesth Analg.* 2004;99:399-408.

Veselis RA, Reinsel RA, Beattie BJ, Mawlawi OR, Feshchenko VA, DiResta GR, Larson SM, Blasberg RG. Midazolam changes cerebral blood flow in discrete brain regions:an H2(15)O positron emission tomography study. *Anaesthesiology.* 1997;87:1106-1117.

Vigand P, Vigand S. *Only the eyes say yes.* Arcade Publishing, New York 2000.

Vogt BA, Finch DM, Olson CR. Functional heterogeneity in cingulate cortex: the anterior executive and posterior evaluative regions. *Cereb Cortex.* 1992;2:435-43.

Volkow ND, Wang GJ, Hitzemann R, Fowler JS, Pappas N, Lowrimore P, Burr G, Pascani K, Overall J, Wolf AP. Depression of thalamic metabolism by lorazepam is associated with sleepiness. *Neuropsychopharmacol.* 1995;12:123-132.

Vuyk J, Engbers FHM, Burm AGL, Vletter AA, Bovill JG. Performance of computer-controlled infusion of propofol: an evaluation of five pharmacokinetic parameter sets. *Anesth Analg.* 1995;81: 1275–82.

Vuyk J, Mertens MJ, Olofsen E, Burm AGL, Bovill JG. Propofol anesthesia and rational opioid selection. *Anesthesiology.* 1997;87:1549-62.

Wade DT, Johnston C. The permanent vegetative state: practical guidance on diagnosis and management. *Br Med J.* 1999; 319:841–44.

White NS, Alkire MT. Impaired thalamocortical connectivity in humans during general-anaesthetic-induced unconsciousness. *Neuroimage.* 2003;19:402-411.

Whyte J, DiPasquale MC. Assessment of vision and visual attention in minimally responsive brain injury patients. *Arch Phys Med Rehabil.* 1995;76:804–10.

Wijdicks EF. The diagnosis of brain death. *N Engl J Med.* 2001;344:1215-21.

Wilson FC, Harpur J, Watson T, Morrow JI. Vegetative state and minimally responsive patients: regional survey, long-term case outcomes and service recommendations. *NeuroRehabilitation* 2002;17:231–36.

Chapter 5

TRANSIENT ALTERATIONS OF CONSCIOUSNESS: EPILEPSY

I felt the sky falling down on earth
– and then it swallowed me.

Fjodor Dostoevskij's decription of his first seizure
to Anna Korvin Krukovskaia and her sister Sonja
(Winter 1865)

5.1. EPILEPSY AND CONSCIOUSNESS

Seizure activity has long been associated with alterations in consciousness. Not surprisingly, the impairment of consciousness is thought to represent a touchstone for the recognition of seizure activity (Gloor 1986). The concept of consciousness is central in epileptology, despite the methodological difficulties concerning its application to the multifaced ictal phenomenology. Generalized seizures are characterized by transient black-outs of consciousness of the self and the environment. Epileptic seizures of focal origin are currently classified according to the status of ictal consciousness, ranging from preserved awareness of the surroundings ("simple" partial seizures) to complete unresponsiveness ("complex" partial seizures). This chapter provides an up-to-date review of the neurological literature on the relationship between epilepsy and consciousness and the neural correlates of ictal loss and impairment of consciousness. We will show that a two-dimensional model (i.e., level *versus* contents of consciousness) fits best with the description of seizure-induced alterations of consciousness, according to the findings of both neuroimaging and electrophysiological studies.

Moreover, the analysis of the general level of awareness and the subjective contents of consciousness is crucial for the understanding of the clinical alterations of the conscious state occurring during the various kinds of epileptic seizures (Johanson et al. 2003). Conversely, the multifaced ictal semiology provides a valuable paradigm to test the reliability of the level-versus-contents model of consciousness.

5.2. CONSCIOUSNESS-AFFECTING SEIZURES

The intimate relationship between conscious staes and epileptic manifestations was officially formalized by the International League Against Epilepsy (ILAE) in 1981, when the revised classification of epileptic seizures recommended that impairment of consciousness be used as the criterion for differentiating simple from complex partial seizures (Commission on Classification and Terminology of the International League Against Epilepsy 1981). Since then, the evaluation of consciousness has been essential to the phenomenological description, diagnosis, and classification of epilepsy (Zappulla 1997).

In addition to complex partial seizures, two other types of seizures are classically known as causing impairment of consciousness: generalized tonic-clonic seizures and childhood absences (Crick et al. 2004; Kalamangalam 2001). As noted before, the difficulties surrounding the criteria for determining impairment of consciousness were resolved by operationally defining consciousness as the patient's responsiveness during the ictal state. Such a use of the concept of consciousness can be misleading, since both generalized and partial seizures entail unresponsiveness during the epileptic discharge, but their effects on the patient's ictal conscious state show significant differences, as a consequence of the different involvement of the neurological substrates (Lee et al. 2002). Generalized seizures are characterized by abnormal electrical activity in both hemispheres and complete loss of consciousness, while complex partial seizures often cause disturbances limited to sensory processes, perception, memory or attention, resulting in motor or sensory aphasia (Kanemoto and Janz 1989), or transient inattention, that are easily misinterpreted as loss of consciousness (Gloor 1986; Luders et al. 1993).

Another controversial portion of the 1981 classification is the inclusion of psychic symptoms, such as ictal affective disturbances and perceptual hallucinations as simple partial seizures, that is partial seizures in which consciousness is preserved (Bromfield 1991; Porter 1991). Diffuse dissatisfaction concerning these ambiguities has been expressed on several occasions through the past few years (Gloor 1986; Luders et al. 1993), so that the inadequacy of the terms "loss" or "impairment" of consciousness in clinical epileptology seems now to be out of question. In 1998, Luders et al. (Luders 1998) proposed a classification of the epileptic seizures based exclusively on ictal semiology. They coined the term "dialeptic seizures" (from the Greek "dialeipein", which means "to interrupt") for ictal episodes in which the main manifestation is alteration of consciousness, irrespective of the ictal and interictal EEG changes. The new term was introduced to differentiate this purely semiological concept from absence seizures (dialeptic seizures with a generalized EEG) and complex partial seizures (dialeptic seizures with a focal ictal EEG), but failed to achieve a widespread acceptance. Eventually, in 2001 the ILAE Task Force on Epilepsy Classification and Terminology proposed a diagnostic scheme for epileptic seizures that substituted the distinction between simple and complex partial seizures with the one between focal sensory seizures with elementary symptoms and focal sensory seizures with experiential symptoms (Engel 2001).

Despite these efforts, ambiguities persist and the assessment of the ictal conscious state is usually left to the observer's subjective interpretation and personal vocabulary. The representation through a bidimensional model helps dissecting the exact nature of the impairment of consciousness, leading to a clear-cut differentiation between seizures that primary affect the level of awareness (generalized seizures) and seizures that specifically alter the contents of the ictal conscious state (focal seizures).

5.3. GENERALIZED SEIZURES AS TRANSIENT BLACK-OUTS

Both primarily and secondarily generalized seizures are invariably associated with a complete and transient loss of consciousness. Consequently, generalized tonic-clonic seizures ("grand mal" epilepsy) and typical childhood absences ("petit mal" epilepsy) are the most common causes of epileptic-induced loss of consciousness (Crick et al. 2004; Kalamangalam 2001). The latter are characterized by rather stereotyped phenomenological features, consisting of a brisk interruption of the patient's behavior, with staring, unresponsiveness, and possible eyelid or mild myoclonic spasms (Avoli et al. 1990). No subjective experience accompanies these relatively frequent seizures, as they entail a sudden "black-out" of both awareness and conscious contents. Several human and animal studies have suggested that absence seizures are generated through abnormal network oscillations involving the cortex of the two hemispheres and the thalamic nuclei, that represent the target of the brainstem reticular activating projections (Snead 1995; Blumenfeld 2002). These oscillations result in the classical EEG pattern of bilateral 3-Hz spike-wave discharges, usually lasting less than 10 seconds (Goldie et al. 1961; Vuilleumier et al. 2000). Human imaging studies have ended in more controversial results, with some studies showing global increases in cerebral blood flow (CBF) (Prevet et al. 1995; Yeni et al. 2000) and others showing variable patterns of increased or decreased brain metabolism (Salek-Haddadi et al. 2002). By combining these data with the results of their studies in animal models, Blumenfeld and Taylor (Crick et al. 2004) formulated the hypothesis that loss of consciousness in absence seizures is due to a disruption of the normal information processing at the level of bilateral association cortices (with a possible predominant role of the frontal neocortex) and related subcortical structures. A similar, yet much more dramatic alteration of consciousness is observed during the course of a generalized convulsive seizure, that can persist for minutes and is invariably accompanied by violent bilateral spasms (Kalamangalam 2001; Porter 1991). The bidimensional model of complete loss of consciousness during a generalized tonic-clonic or absence seizure is shown in Figure 5.1. Notably, both the level and the contents of the conscious state are virtually absent.

Studies based on electrophysiological, blood flow, and metabolic mapping suggest that the entire brain may be homogeneously involved in primary generalized tonic-clonic seizures (Lee et al. 2002; Fiset et al. 1999). However, a recent single photon emission computed tomography (SPECT) ictal-interictal imaging study reported that the regions most intensely involved by CBF increase were bilateral frontal and parietal association cortices, together with thalamus and upper brainstem (Crick et al. 2004). Again, a temporarily low functional connectivity between bilateral cortical regions, and between thalamus and cortex seem to be the main mechanism accounting for the loss of consciousness. Accordingly to this model, Baars et al. (Baars et al. 2003) have recently compared the brain mechanisms of four unconscious states that are causally very different from each other: deep sleep, coma/vegetative states, epileptic loss of consciousness, and drug-induced general anesthesia. Despite their different aetiologies, all these conditions present as major common features widely synchronized slow waveforms that take the place of the fast and flexible interactions needed for conscious functions, and a temporarily blocked functional connectivity, both cortico-cortical and thalamo-cortical.

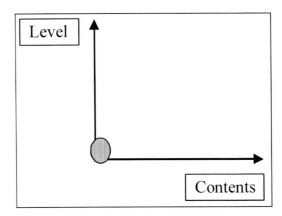

Figure 5.1. Bidimensional model of the loss of consciousness during a generalized seizure. Both the level of arousal and the contents of conscious experience are virtually absent. [reprinted from Cavanna AE, Mula M, Monaco F. Epilepsy and Consciousness. In: Holloway KJ (Ed) New research on epilepsy and behavior. New York: Nova Publishers; 2007].

Generalized epileptic seizures accompanied by complete, albeit short-lasting loss of consciousness, can also be induced artificially by applying electric currents (70 to 600 volts from 0.5 to 4 seconds) through the scalp of a subject. The electric current can be applied by positioning a couple of electrodes on the head, either unilaterally or bilaterally. This technique, which is called electroconvulsive therapy (ECT), was introduced as a treatment for schizophrenia in the 1930s, and since then became a feasible treatment option for a wide range of patients with psychiatric disorders. The introduction of antipsychotic and antidepressant pharmacotherapy around the 1950s and the 1960s led to a decline of the clinical use of ECT, but it has maintained a relatively important place in psychiatry, mainly as a treatment for drug-resistant major depression (Fink 2001). In a review of the literature on the well-known ECT complication of epilepsy, Devinsky and Duchowny (1983) calculated that the age-adjusted incidence of new seizures after ECT was fivefold greater than the incidence found in non-psychiatric populations.

Quite recently, studies of patients with generalized spike-wave activity have achieved excellent standards of spatial and temporal resolution by coupling functional magnetic resonance imaging (fMRI) with simultaneous EEG recordings (Gotman et al. 2006; Laufs et al. 2006). Quite interestingly, preliminary EEG-fMRI findings confirmed that generalized seizures may selectively involve certain networks, while sparing others. In particular, they demonstrated bilateral thalamic activation and cortical signal decrease in a characteristic distribution of association areas that are most active during conscious rest, i.e. prefrontal, lateral parietal and midline precuneus/posterior cingulate cortex. According to the "default mode of brain function" hypothesis, these areas show transient deactivations whenever healthy subjects are engaged in non-self referential cognitive tasks and in conditions of strongly reduced vigilance, such as deep sleep, coma/vegetative states, and drug-induced general anesthesia (Cavanna and Trimble 2006). EEG-fMRI studies of impaired consciousness in generalized seizures provide further evidence that default mode areas likely represent a key part of the neural network subserving the level of general awareness.

5.4. PARTIAL SEIZURES AND EXPERIENTIAL PHENOMENA

Focal epileptic seizures originate in specific parts of the cortex and either remain confined to those areas or spread to other parts of the brain. The clinical manifestations of the seizures are related to the area of the cortex in which the seizures start, how widely they are propagated and how long they last (Daly 1975; Yamauchi 1998). Since the early observations of the British neurologist John Hughlings-Jackson (1835-1911), it is clear that local epileptic activity arising from the temporal lobe often creates experiential events in the patient's mind. Hughlings-Jackson made the first systematic study of these conscious contents and wrote of "psychical states which are much more elaborate than crude sensations" (Hughlings-Jackson 1880). Such manifestations of temporal lobe epilepsy are still among the most fascinating and poorly understood neurological phenomena.

Experiential phenomena are usually brief and coincide with the onset of a complex partial seizure. Sometimes they are followed by automatisms, stereotyped behavioral patterns (e.g. smacking, chewing, etc.) that occur in an environment of altered responsiveness and amnesia for the activity (Daly 1975; Theodore et al. 1983; Marks and Laxer 1998).

A common presentation of experiential phenomena is within the context of an epileptic aura, a subjective ictal phenomenon that may precede an observable seizure (Lennox and Cobb 1933; Taylor and Lochery 1987). Both experiential sensory seizures and auras can include affective, mnemonic, or composite perceptual phenomena (Devinsky and Luciano 1991; Mula et al. 2003). The latter are complex hallucinations and illusions involving all sensory systems, but most commonly the visual or auditory modalities (Gloor 1990). Patients may see complex scenes, faces, or hear voices or segments of music being played; the content of these hallucinations usually appears familiar to them, although they may not always be able to identify it specifically. However, they are usually struck by the illusionary nature of their experience (Rainville et al. 2002; Devinsky and Luciano 1991).

Memory phenomena of two kinds occur, in particular in temporal lobe seizures. First, there may be actual recall of past event or situation, usually more vivid and intrusive than a commonplace recollection (Luders et al. 1993; Rainville et al. 2002). Secondly, there may be a feeling of recognition, of familiarity or reminiscence. If the feeling of familiarity occurs in isolation, it is often inappropriately attached to the present, creating the illusion that the present is like the re-enactment of a past situation or event, the so-called "déjà-vu" (Sno and Linszen 1990; Bancaud et al. 1994).

The affective components of experiential phenomena include subjective feelings of fear, euphoria, guilt, depression, sadness, joy, sexual excitement, pleasure and (rarely) anger (Williams 1956; Janszy et al. 2004). An ictal emotional experience usually accompanies the contents of perceptual hallucinations or memory recall, but can also occur in isolation, apparently unexplained, yet deeply embedded in the patient's personal life (Devinsky and Luciano 1991; Mula et al. 2003). Hughlings-Jackson gave this isolated psychic phenomenon different labels, such as "dreamy state", "intellectual aura", "voluminous" mental state, and "over-consciousness" (Hughlings-Jackson 1880; Alvarez-Silva et al. 2006). It usually includes symptoms of depersonalisation (altered sense of self) and derealization (altered experience of the external world), and delusional features are not uncommon (Devinsky and Luciano 1991; Fried 1997). Mystical and religious feelings have been occasionally reported (Cirignotta et al. 1980; Hansen and Brodtkorb 2003). These rare experiences were beautifully described by one of the most talented and prolific authors affected by epilepsy, Fyodor Dostoyevsky (Figure 5.2) (Hughes 2005).

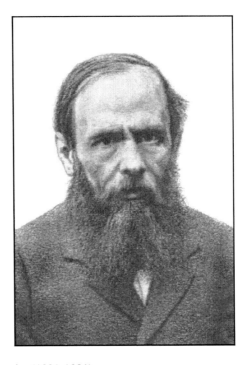

Figure 5.2. Fyodor Dostoyevsky (1821-1881).

Dostoyevsky used to include an epileptic character in most of his novels, as Prince Myshkin in "The Idiot" (1868), who experiences the following ecstatic feelings during an epileptic aura: "his sensation of being alive and his awareness increased tenfold… his mind and heart were flooded by a dazzling light… culminating in a great calm, full of serene and harmonious joy and hope, full of understanding and knowledge of the final cause" (Dostoyevsky 1955).

It seems reasonable to assume that he was describing his own mystical experience in the context of an epileptic aura. However, others have suggested that it was his literary genius that ascribed this experience to the epilepsy, and that it did not occur in his aura but independently of a seizure.

In any event, positive experiences as part of the temporal lobe aura are extremely rare. In Gower's 1881 study of 505 epileptic auras only 3% were said to be emotional, and none positive. In the Lennox (1960) study of 1017 auras, only 9 were said to be pleasant (0.9%) and of these, "only a few showed positive pleasure." Penfield and Kristiansen (1951) cite only one case of an aura with a pleasant sensation, followed by an epigastric feeling of discomfort. However, in 1982 Cirignotta published an account of a patient who had just such an aura as that described by Dostoevsky before a temporal lobe seizure arising in his right temporal lobe. There is thus undoubted scientific evidence that such auras (alterations of the contents of consciousness) do exist prior to a seizure and that they are likely to be associated with the right temporal structures. Overall, these findings suggest a common link between temporal lobe function and mystical experience.

5.4.1. Penfield's Experiments

Penfield (Penfield 1938) made the important discovery that these mental phenomena could be reproduced by electrical stimulation of the temporal lobe in epileptic patients during surgical procedures.

Penfield's procedure involved an ingenious way of finding out which areas of a patient's brain were those that were prone to cause epileptic seizures. At first, he observed that, shortly before a seizure occurred, the person suffering from epilepsy would often report suffering hallucinations, or experiencing a disgusting smell, or being overcome by a strange feeling (the epileptic aura). Penfield hypothesized that he could isolate the disease-damaged areas, and so those areas which were the likely cause of future epileptic seizures, by introducing into those areas an electrical current that mimicked to a certain extent the brain's own electrical activity. If the result was an epileptic aura, he knew that he had located the right areas. Penfield needed the patient to be awake during this period of electrical probing, so that she could report if and when the hallucinations or strange smells or feelings occurred. As the brain can notoriously be probed with electrodes without a patient suffering any pain, most patients readily agreed to this probing. Penfield reported that the results of his electrical probings, especially in the area of the temporal lobes, astonished even himself. He mentioned some of his cases in his Sherrington Lectures delivered at the University of Liverpool in January 1957, and subsequently published as The Excitable Cortex in Conscious Man (1958). One of the early cases in 1938 was that of M.G., a 16 years old Canadian woman who complained of seizures that were ushered in by hearing a song, a lullaby her mother had often sung to her, "Hush a bye, my baby...". In addition to this song, there was often what she called a 'dream' in this stage of her attacks, during which she would be in church or in the convent. During the operation, when the superior gyrus of the right temporal lobe was stimulated, she gave a little exclamation. Then after the electrode had been withdrawn she said, "I had a dream. I wasn't here". After talking with her for a little while, the electrode was reapplied at the same point without her knowledge. She broke off suddenly and said, "I hear people coming in". Then she added, "I hear music now, a funny little piece". The electrode was kept in place and she became more talkative, saying that the music she was hearing was something she had heard on the radio. It was the song her mother had sung. A few minutes later, the same point was stimulated, again without warning her. She said, "Another dream. People coming in...". Penfield had succeeded in electrical reproduction of the hallucination drawn from her past experience which had, for years, introduced her epileptic seizures. He found that the "hallucinations" were made up of elements from the individual's past experiences. In fact, the subjects, while conscious of themselves as in the present, and in the clinic, were not so much recalling, as actually reliving, in a very vivid and somehow fractured way, certain past experiences. That is why they seemed invariably to think of them as dreams. Furthermore, in normal circumstances the patients were not able to relive these past experiences in this way. Apparently, Penfield had tapped directly into the hidden world of lived past experiences. He concluded that local neuronal activity at the level of an epileptogenic zone can produce higher order experiences, and called them "experiential phenomena", because they had a compelling immediacy similar to or sometimes more vivid than the patient's recall of his own past experiences. While these responses were originally described following stimulation of the temporal neocortex, subsequent studies suggested that they are more prevalent during stimulation of the limbic components of the medial temporal lobe, particularly the amygdala (Rainville et al. 2002; Halgren et al. 1978).

5.4.2. The Neural Correlates of Epileptic Qualia

In addition to their clinical significance (Taylor and Lochery 1987; Palmini and Gloor 1992; Lux et al. 2002), seizure-induced experiential phenomena raise interesting questions concerning brain mechanisms involved in the production of some the most familiar human experiences, that the current philosophical jargon refers to as phenomenal qualia (Kalamangalam 2001) (see chapter 1). Clearly, the detailed investigation of the neural processes taking place at the level of the limbic structures of medial temporal lobe during complex partial seizures, provides interesting avenues and precious insights for the ultimate search of the neural correlates of qualia. As mentioned before, psychic or experiential phenomena that involve perceptual, mnemonic, and affective processes can be elicited by medial temporal lobe seizures, discharges, and stimulation. For example, the activation of the amygdala and other limbic structures is responsible for the affective component of experiential phenomena (Rainville et al. 2002; Halgren et al. 1978; Gloor 1991; Van Paesschen et al. 2001). Therefore, focal seizures are thought to modulate the contents of ictal conscious state in medial temporal lobe epilepsy. Figure 5.3 shows the bidimensional model of altered conscious states during a focal seizure/aura with experiential symptoms. The level of arousal presents with a huge variability, yet the contents of consciousness are highly vivid, characterized by seizure-induced experiential phenomena or emotional qualia. The conceptual validity of this dissociation between consciousness level and content is highlighted by the fact that occasional seizures have been recorded in which the patient is normally responsive even though experiencing psychic symptoms (Porter 1991).

The neurobiological changes associated to complex partial seizures have also been recently addressed by functional imaging studies. Interictal and ictal SPECT with early injection during complex partial seizures in patients with hippocampal sclerosis showed ictal hyperperfusion in the temporal lobe ipsilateral to the seizure focus, along with ipsilateral middle frontal and precentral gyrus and both occipital lobes. Conversely, the frontal lobes, contralateral posterior cerebellum and ipsilateral precuneus showed hypoperfusion (Van Paesschen et al. 2003). In another SPECT ictal-interictal study in patients with surgically confirmed mesial temporal sclerosis, Blumenfeld et al. (2004a) analysed ictal CBF changes, while performing continuous video/EEG monitoring. They found that temporal lobe seizures associated with loss of consciousness (complex partial seizures) produced CBF increases in the temporal lobe, followed by increases in bilateral midline subcortical structures, including the mediodorsal thalamus and upper brainstem. These changes were accompanied by marked bilateral hypometabolism in the frontal and parietal association cortices (lateral prefrontal, anterior cingulate, orbital frontal, and lateral parietal cortex). In contrast, temporal lobe seizures in which consciousness was spared (simple partial seizures) were associated with more limited changes, mainly confined to the temporal lobe, and were not accompanied by such widespread impaired function of the fronto-parietal association cortices. Intracranial EEG recordings from temporal lobe seizures accompanied by impaired responsiveness confirmed the profound slowing in bilateral frontal and parietal association cortices, which is particularly severe in the late ictal phase and extends to the early post-ictal period (Blumenfeld et al. 2004b).

These findings are consistent with Norden and Blumenfeld's "network inhibition hypothesis", according to which focal seizures arising in the medial temporal lobe spread to subcortical structures (medial diencephalon and pontomesencephalic reticular formation) and disrupt their activating function, secondarily leading to widespread inhibition of nonseizing regions of the frontal and parietal association cortex (Norden and Blumenfeld 2002). The fronto-parietal network inhibition may ultimately be responsible for the impaired level of consciousness reported in the late ictal and immediate post-ictal phase of some complex partial seizures. Such intriguing, yet sophisticated, model of selective association cortex inhibition by a focal cortical seizure is gradually replacing the long-lasting concept of critical mass of cerebral tissue involved in seizure spread to cause impairment of consciousness.

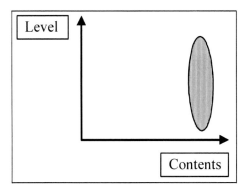

Figure 5.3. Bidimensional model of altered conscious states during a focal seizure with experiential symptoms. The level of arousal displays a wide range of degrees, while the contents of consciousness are almost constantly vivid. [reprinted from Cavanna AE, Mula M, Monaco F. Epilepsy and Consciousness. In: Holloway KJ (Ed) New research on epilepsy and behavior. New York: Nova Publishers; 2007].

5.5. LIMBIC STATUS EPILEPTICUS: THE "ZOMBIE STATE"

During limbic status epilepticus – formerly called "psychomotor status", or "dialeptic status" in the semiological seizure classification – patients sometimes pose considerable problems for the observer. Penfield (1975) describes epileptic patients who are "totally unconscious", but nonetheless continue their activities of walking in a crowded street or driving home or playing a piano piece even for hours, but in a sort of inflexible and uncreative way. They seem capable of sidestepping obstacles in the environment, grasp objects, and sometimes respond to movement and speech – yet, they are not aware of their purposeful actions. More recently, Fried (1997) reported the analogous case of a patient whose seizures occurred while he was riding his bicycle to work. After setting out for work, he would occasionally find himself riding back home. Apparently, during his seizures he was able to turn around and operate a bicycle. Koch and Crick (2001) called these seemingly automatic activities "zombie modes". In philosophy of mind, zombies are conceived as beings whose behavior is utterly indistinguishable from that of normal humans, but who have no "inner life" at all. In other words, philosophical zombies lack phenomenal qualia, and therefore do not experience subjective feelings (Chalmers 1996; Skokowski 2002).

In everyday life, such zombie modes are involved in a good portion of our behavior, but they act in parallel with our conscious attention focusing elsewhere. For instance, when we are driving the car "on automatic pilot" while having a conversation, we are not paying much attention to the details of the road and the traffic. But it is simply not true that we are totally unconscious of these phenomena: otherwise, there would be a car crash. Similarly, it has to be postulated that during limbic status epilepticus, although unresponsive and presumably devoid of any conscious content, some patients do retain a basic level of consciousness. Philosopher of mind John Searle, while stressing the importance of these cases for consciousness studies, claims that these patients temporarily lack the function of "phenomenal" consciousness (qualia) and retain "cognitive" consciousness, that allows them to display a zombie-like behavior (Searle 1992).

This scenario is represented in Figure 5.4, showing the bidimensional model of altered conscious states during limbic status epilepticus. The lack of any subjective experience is accompanied by a degree of awareness of the external environment, resulting in a rather automatic, zombie-like behavior.

An alternative explanation for this interesting phenomenon focuses on the temporary impairment of selective attention. Attention has been regarded as a control process in relationship to consciousness (Maquet 2000). Some patients reported being totally absorbed in a compelling seizure-induced experiential phenomenon. When asked why they did not reply to the examiner's questions during the episode, these patients usually reply that they "were there", indicating their complete absorption in the experience (Gloor 1986).

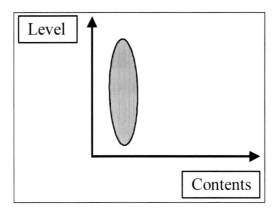

Figure 5.4. Bidimensional model of altered conscious states during a limbic status epilepticus. The level of arousal and responsiveness can vary, but no subjective experiences are present ("zombie-like behavior"). [reprinted from Cavanna AE, Mula M, Monaco F. Epilepsy and Consciousness. In: Holloway KJ (Ed) New research on epilepsy and behavior. New York: Nova Publishers; 2007].

In a recent analysis of 40 descriptions of subjective experiences during complex partial seizures, Johanson and colleagues (Johanson et al. 2003) identified an impairment of the voluntary control of attention as a constant feature of the seizures. Attention was very strongly affected/influenced during the seizures, in a way that could be described as an impairment of voluntary control of attention ("forced attention"). They called this phenomenon "forced attention", because it included the narrowing of the focus of attention and the absence of the voluntary control of the direction of attention. Although largely underrecognized, forced attention seems to characterize the early stage of the seizure and appears to be a fairly common element in the subjective experience of the seizure; it was reported by all subjects enrolled in the study. The neurophysiological explanation for this ictal phenomenon has been suggested to be the spreading of pathological electrophysiological discharges to the frontal networks involved in attentional control (Goode et al. 1970).

These cases show significant similarities to the subjects described by Penfield as being somewhat aware of their environment, yet totally caught by the vividness of the emotional experiences induced by the electrical stimulation of the temporal lobe. Penfield's conclusion was that these patients were simultaneously experiencing "two separate streams of consciousness" (Penfield 1968). Interestingly, a very similar concept dates back to Hughlings-Jackson, who called the symptoms of the "dreamy state" a "double consciousness" (Taylor 1958). In this state, patients were vaguely aware of ongoing events (one consciousness), but were preoccupied with the intrusion of an "all knowing" or "familiar" feeling (a second consciousness). Hughlings-Jackson's well-known description of the case of Dr. Z (Taylor 1980) could be interpreted as just another example of a zombie-like behavior displayed by a physician suffering from a seizure while attending a patient. Quite surprisingly, the "double consciousness" he experienced didn't prevent him from giving the right diagnosis of "pneumonia of the left base", as he was later able to ascertain from his notes. Dr. Z's postmortem examination, in which Hughlings-Jackson himself participated, revealed a "very small patch of softening in the left uncinate gyrus" (Hogan and Kaiboriboon 2003).

5.6. THE ASSESSMENT OF CONSCIOUSNESS IN TEMPORAL LOBE EPILEPSY

The bidimensional model (level *versus* contents) for the description of seizure-induced alterations of consciousness as outlined in this chapter has been recently tested in a clinical setting. Quite recently, the authors of this volume evaluated 41 seizure descriptions from 33 consecutive patients referred to their Epilepsy Unit with a diagnosis of temporal lobe epilepsy (TLE) (Monaco et al. 2006). Accurate descriptions of ictal semiology and subjective experiences were collected by means of semistructured clinical interviews with patients and reliable witnesses. All subjects underwent psychometric assessment using the Beck Depression Inventory (BDI) (Beck et al. 1961), the State-Trait Anxiety Inventory (STAI) (Spielberger et al. 1970), and the Ictal Consciousness Inventory (ICI), a new 20-item questionnaire specifically developed to assess (1) the level of general awareness/responsiveness and (2) the "vividness" of ictal experiential phenomena (Table 5.1).

Table 5.1. The ICI (Ictal Consciousness Inventory)

During the seizure were you...	
1. aware of what was happening to you?	0 - 1 - 2
2. aware of your surroundings?	0 - 1 - 2
3. aware of the time passing by?	0 - 1 - 2
4. aware of the presence of anyone around you?	0 - 1 - 2
5. able to understand other people's words?	0 - 1 - 2
6. able to reply to other people's words (e.g. *What's wrong with you?*)?	0 - 1 - 2
7. able to obey other people's commands (e.g. *Sit down!*)?	0 - 1 - 2
8. able to control the direction of your gaze?	0 - 1 - 2
9. able to focus your attention?	0 - 1 - 2
10. able to take any initiative?	0 - 1 - 2
During the seizure did you...	
11. feel like you were in a dream?	0 - 1 - 2
12. feel like you were in an unusually familiar place?	0 - 1 - 2
13. feel that things around you were unknown?	0 - 1 - 2
14. feel that everything was in slow motion or sped up?	0 - 1 - 2
15. feel the presence of another person who was not there?	0 - 1 - 2
16. see or hear things that were not real?	0 - 1 - 2
17. see people/objects changing shape?	0 - 1 - 2
18. experience flashbacks or memories of past events (as though you were reliving the past)?	0 - 1 - 2
19. experience unpleasant emotions (e.g. fear, sadness, anger)?	0 - 1 - 2
20. experience pleasant emotions (e.g. joy, happiness, pleasure)?	0 - 1 - 2

Please answer the following questions by referring to a single seizure, witnessed by another person.
Answers: 0 = no; 1 = yes, a bit (yes, vaguely); 2 = yes, much (yes, clearly).

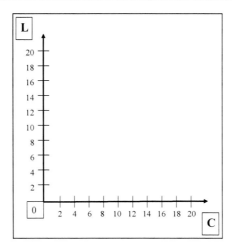

The first ten questions of the ICI concern the level of consciousness and assess reflective consciousness; general awareness of time, place, and other people's presence; understanding of other people's words; verbal and nonverbal responsiveness; gaze control; forced attention; voluntary initiative. On the other hand, items 11-20 refer to the contents of consciousness and assess the following subjective experiences: dreamy states; derealization symptoms (regarding time and space); feeling of the presence of an absent person; illusions; hallucinations; déjà vu/vécu; unpleasant and pleasant ictal emotions. Each item is rated by the subject on a 0-2 likert scale, and the inventory yields an overall score (range 0-40) and two subscores for level (L) and contents (C) of ictal consciousness (range 0-20).

The preliminary quantification of both objective and subjective features of ictal consciousness in patients with TLE showed that the vast majority (>80%) of seizures involving altered conscious experiences are accompanied by a degree of responsiveness and/or retained awareness of the surroundings. Each seizure description could be plotted into a biaxial diagram according to ICI subscores for level and contents of ictal consciousness (see Table 1). L and C subscores showed a positive correlation, however the two dimensions were not associated with age at onset, duration of disease, seizure frequency, or localisation of EEG focus. Interestingly, only C subscores correlated significantly with affective psychopathology, as assessed by supra-threshold BDI and STAI scores. In other words, the presence of emotionally vivid experiential phenomena was selectively associated with comorbid mood and anxiety disorders. These findings support previous studies showing that temporolimbic structures could represent a common substrate for ictal emotional experiences and interictal affective disturbances in patients with TLE (Reynders et al. 2005; Mula et al. 2006). Moreover, the preliminary results of this phenomenological investigation represent the first step toward the development of a systematic approach for the combined assessment of the level of awareness and the subjective contents of consciousness during epileptic seizures of temporal lobe origin, and the identification of putative psychopathological correlations.

5.7. A WINDOW OVER THE TWO DIMENSIONS OF CONSCIOUSNESS

In summary, both the level of awareness and the contents of mental states are affected by epileptic seizures. Generalized tonic-clonic and absence seizures primarily impair the level of consciousness ("black-out"), while focal seizures mainly alter the patient's private experiences. Sometimes the changes in the conscious state encompass both the level and the contents, in a very articulate and entangled way, as in complex partial seizures of temporal lobe origin. In this respect, a bidimensional model displaying the level and the contents of consciousness in two separate axes could prove to be highly valuable in assessing both the quantitative and qualitative changes that characterize the ictal conscious state. Table 5.2 summarizes the pattern of alterations of the level and contents of consciousness in the ictal semeiologies described in this chapter, thus providing the conceptual framework for plotting consciousness-affecting seizures into the biaxial diagram.

Ictal neurophysiological and imaging findings provide a sound basis for the development of such a model, as different neural mechanisms have been shown to underlie the level and the content of consciousness. As for determining the level of awareness, a crucial role seems to be played by either primitive (in generalized seizures) or secondary (in focal seizures) involvement of subcortical structures. On the other hand, the qualitative features of experiential phenomena – arguably the most precise neuropathological correlate of the philosophical concept of qualia – are mainly the expression of the activity of limbic components of the temporal lobe. A systematic analysis of such experiential phenomena should be included in a complete diagnostic protocol for epilepsy, in order to achieve a better understanding of the patient's subjective ictal experience.

Table 5.2. Summary of the possible alterations in the cardinal parameters of the bidimensional model (level and contents of the ictal conscious state) in the main seizure types affecting consciousness

Seizure	Level of consciousness	Contents of consciousness
Generalized tonic-clonic	↓	↓
Absence	↓	↓
Focal, experiential type	↓↑	↑
Limbic status	↓↑	↓

Overall, epilepsy represents a privileged window into the neural bases of consciousness, as the investigation of this disorder can reveal precious insights into altered conscious states. On the other hand, the confounding clinical evaluation of ictal consciousness could benefit from the neurobiological and philosophical tools provided by the multidisciplinary consciousness studies. Further investigations of the neural correlates of seizure-induced qualitative experiences (qualia) may contribute to shedding light on some of the unanswered questions concerning the brain mechanisms involved in the production of human conscious experiences.

5.8. REFERENCES

Alvarez-Silva S, Alvarez-Silva I, Alvarez-Rodriguez J, Perez-Echeverria MJ, Campayo-Martinez A, Rodriguez-Fernandez FL. Epileptic consciousness: concept and meaning of aura. *Epilepsy Behav.* 2006;8:527-33.

Avoli M, Gloor P, Kostopoulos G, Naquet T, editors. *Generalized epilepsy.* Birkhauser, Boston 1990.

Baars B, Ramsoy TZ, Laureys S. Brain, conscious experience and the observing self. *Trends Neurosci.* 2003;26:671-5.

Bancaud J, Brunet-Bourgin F, Chanvel P, Hargren E. Anatomical origin of déjà vu and vivid "memories" in human temporal lobe epilepsy. *Brain.* 1994;117:71-91.

Banks WP. How much work a quale can do? *Conscious Cogn.* 1996;5:368-80.

Beck AT, Ward CH, Mendelson M, Mock J, Erbaugh J. An inventory for measuring depression. *Arch Gen Psychiatry.* 1961;4:561-71.

Block N. Qualia. In: Gregory R, editor. *The Oxford companion to the mind.* Oxford University Press, Oxford 2004:785-9.

Blumenfeld H, McCormick DA. Corticothalamic inputs control the pattern of activity generated in thalamocortical networks. *J Neurosci.* 2000;20:5153-62.

Blumenfeld H, McNally KA, Vanderhill SD, Paige AL, Chung R, Davis K, Norden AD, Stokking R, Studholme C, Novotny EJ Jr, Zubal IG, Spencer SS. Positive and negative network correlations in temporal lobe epilepsy. *Cereb Cortex.* 2004a;14:892-902.

Blumenfeld H, Rivera M, McNally KA, Davis K, Spencer DD, Spencer SS. Ictal neocortical slowing in temporal lobe epilepsy. *Neurology.* 2004b;63:1015-21.

Blumenfeld H. The thalamus and seizures. *Arch Neurol.* 2002;59:135-37.

Bromfield EB. Somatosensory, special sensory, and autonomic phenomena in seizures. *Semin Neurol.* 1991;11:91-9.

Cavanna AE, Trimble MR. The precuneus: a review of its functional anatomy and behavioural correlates. *Brain.* 2006;129:564-83.

Chalmers D. *The conscious mind: in search of a fundamental theory.* Oxford University Press, Oxford 1996.

Cirignotta F, Todesco CV, Lugaresi E. Temporal lobe epilepsy with ecstatic seizures (so-called Dostoevsky epilepsy). *Epilepsia.* 1980;21:705-10.

Commission on Classification and Terminology of the International League Against Epilepsy. Proposal for revised clinical and electroencephalographic classification of seizures. *Epilepsia.* 1981;22:489-501.

Crick F, Koch C, Kreiman G, Fried I. Consciousness and neurosurgery. *Neurosurgery.* 2004;55:273-82.

Daly DD. Ictal affect. *Am J Psychiatry.* 1958;115:97-108.

Daly DD. Ictal clinical manifestations of complex partial seizures. *Adv Neurol.* 1975;11:57-83.

Dennett D. Quining qualia. In: Marcel AJ, Bisiach E, editors. *Consciousness in contemporary science.* Clarendon Press, Oxford 1988:42-77.

Devinsky O, Duchowny MS. Seizures after convulsive therapy: a retrospective case survey. *Neurology.* 1983;33:921-5.

Devinsky O, Luciano D. Psychic phenomena in partial seizures. *Semin Neurol.* 1991;11:100-9.

Dostoyevsky FM. The idiot. Penguin Books, London 1955 [Translation of 1869 ed. by Magarshack D].

Engel J Jr. A proposed diagnostic scheme for people with epileptic seizures and with epilepsy: report of the ILAE Task Force on Classification and Terminology. *Epilepsia.* 2001;42:796-803.

Feichtinger M, Pauli E, Schafer I, Eberhardt KW, Tomandl B, Huk J, Stefan H. Ictal fear in temporal lobe epilepsy. *Arch Neurol.* 2001;58:771-7.

Fink M. Convulsive therapy: a review of the first 55 years. *J Affect Dis.* 2001;63:1-15.

Fiset P, Paus T, Daloze T, Plourde G, Meuret P, Bonhomme V, Hajj-Ali N, Backman SB, Evans AC. Brain mechanisms of propofol-induced loss of consciousness. *J Neurosci.* 1999;19:5506-13.

Fish DR, Gloor P, Querney FL, Olivier A. Clinical responses to electrical brain stimulation of the temporal and frontal lobes in patients with epilepsy. *Brain.* 1993;116:397-414.

Fried I. Auras and experiential responses arising in the temporal lobe. *J Neuropsychiatry Clin Neurosci.* 1997;9:420-8.

Gloor P. Consciousness as a neurological concept in epileptology: a critical review. *Epilepsia.* 1986;27(Suppl 2):14-26.

Gloor P. Experiential phenomena of temporal lobe epilepsy: facts and hypotheses. *Brain.* 1990;113:1673-94.

Gloor P. Neurobiological substrates of ictal behavioral changes. *Adv Neurol.* 1991;55:1-34.

Gloor P. *The temporal lobe and limbic system.* Oxford University Press, new York 1997.

Goldie L, Green JM. Spike and wave discharges and alterations of conscious awareness. *Nature.* 1961;191:200-1.

Goode DJ, Penry JK, Dreifuss FE. Effects of paroxysmal spike-wave on continuous visual-motor performance. *Epilepsia.* 1970;11:241-54.

Gotman J, Grova C, Bagshaw A, Kobayashi E, Aghakhani Y, Dubeau F. Generalized epileptic discharges show thalamocortical activation and suspension of the default state of the brain. *Proc Natl Acad Sci.* 2006;102:15236-40.

Gray J. How are qualia coupled to functions? *Trends Cogn Sci.* 2003;7:192-4.

Gupta AK, Jeavons PM, Hughes RC, Covanis A. Aura in temporal lobe epilepsy: clinical and electroencephalographic correlation. *J Neurol Neurosurg Psychiatry.* 1983;46:1079-83.

Halgren E, Walter RD, Cherlow DG, Crandall PH. Mental phenomena evoked by electrical stimulation of the human hippocampal formation and amygdala. *Brain.* 1978;101:83-117.

Hansen BA, Brodtkorb E. Partial epilepsy with "ecstatic" seizures. *Epilepsy Behav.* 2003;4:667-73.

Hogan RE, Kaiboriboon K. The "dreamy state": John Hughlings-Jackson's ideas of epilepsy and consciousness. *Am J Psychiatry.* 2003;160:1740-7.

Hughes JR. The idiosyncratic aspects of the epilepsy of Fyodor Dostoevsky. *Epilepsy Behav.* 2005;7:531-8.

Hughlings-Jackson J. On a particular variety of epilepsy ("intellectual aura"), one case with symptoms of organic brain disease. *Brain.* 1888;11:179-207.

Hughlings-Jackson J. On right or left-sided spasms at the onset of epileptic paroxysms, and on crude sensation warnings and elaborate mental states. *Brain.* 1880;3:192-206.

Janszky J, Ebner A, Szupera Z, Schulz R, Hollo A, Szucs A, Clemens B. Orgasmic aura: a report of seven cases. *Seizure.* 2004;13:441-4.

Johanson M, Revonsuo A, Chaplin J, Wedlund JE. Level and contents of consciousness in connection with partial epileptic seizures. *Epilepsy Behav.* 2003;4:279-85.

Kalamangalam GP. Epilepsy and the physical basis of consciousness. *Seizure.* 2001;10:484-91.

Kanemoto K, Janz D. The temporal sequence of aura sensations in patients with complex focal seizures with particular attention to ictal aphasia. *J Neurol Neurosurg Psychiatry.* 1989;52:52-56.

Kanemoto K. Epilepsy and recursive consciousness with special attention to Jackson's theory of consciousness. *Epilepsia.* 1998;39:11-5.

Koch C, Crick FC. The zombie within. *Nature.* 2001;411:893.

Kostopoulos GK. Involvement of the thalamocortical system in epileptic loss of consciousness. *Epilepsia.* 2001;42:13-9.

Laufs H, Lengler U, Hamandi K, Kleinschmidt A, Krakow K. Linking generalized spike-and-wave discharges and resting state brain activity by using EEG/fMRI in a patient with absence seizures. *Epilepsia.* 2006;47:444-8.

Lee KH, Meador KJ, Park YD, King DW, Murro AM, Pillai JJ, Kaminski RJ. Pathophysiology of altered consciousness during seizures: subtraction SPECT study. *Neurology.* 2002;59:841-6.

Lennox WG, Cobb S. Aura in epilepsy: a statistical review of 1359 cases. *Arch Neurol.* 1933;30:374-87.

Lewis D. Should a materialist believe in qualia? *Australas J Philos.* 1995;73:140-4.

Luders H, Acharya J, Baumgartner C, Benbadis S, Bleasel A, Burgess R, Dinner DS, Ebner A, Foldvary N, Geller E, Hamer H, Holthausen H, Kotagal P, Morris H, Meencke HJ, Noachtar S, Rosenow F, Sakamoto A, Steinhoff BJ, Tuxhorn I, Wyllie E. Semiological seizure classification. *Epilepsia.* 1998;39:1006-13.

Luders HO, Burgess R, Noachtar S. Expanding the international classification of seizures to provide localization information. *Neurology.* 1993;43:1650-5.

Lux S, Kurthen M, Helmstaedter C, Hartje W, Reuber M, Elger CE. The localizing value of ictal consciousness and its constituent functions. A video-EEG study in patients with focal epilepsy. *Brain.* 2002;125:2691-8.

Maquet P. Functional neuroimaging of normal human sleep by positron emission tomography. *J Sleep Res.* 2000; 9:207-31.

Marks WJ, Laxer KD. Semiology of temporal lobe seizures: value in lateralizing the seizure focus. *Epilepsia.* 1998;39:721-6.

Mayanagi Y, Watanabe E, Kaneko Y. Mesial temporal lobe epilepsy: clinical features and seizure mechanism. *Epilepsia.* 1996;37(Suppl. 3):57-60.

Monaco F, Mula M, Collimedaglia L, Barbagli D, Tota G, Cantello R, O'Callaghan P, Cavanna AE. Level and contents of ictal consciousness in temporal lobe epilepsy. *Epilepsia.* 2006;47(Suppl. 3):23.

Mula M, Cavanna A, Collimedaglia L, Barbagli D, Magli E, Monaco F. The role of aura in psychopathology and dissociative experiences in epilepsy. *J Neuropsy Clin Neurosci.* 2006 18:536-42.

Mula M, Trimble MR, Monaco F. Psychopathology in epilepsy: the peri-ictal phenomena. *Ital J Psychopathol.* 2003;9:400-4.

Nagel T. What is it like to be a bat? In: *Mortal questions.* Cambridge University Press, Cambridge 1979:165-80.

Naito H, Matsui N. Temporal lobe epilepsy with ictal ecstatic state and interictal behavior of hypergraphia. *J Nerv Ment Dis.* 1988;176:123-4.

Norden AD, Blumenfeld H. The role of subcortical structures in human epilepsy. *Epilepsy Behav.* 2002;3:219-31.

Palmini A, Gloor G. The localizing value of auras in partial seizures: a prospective and retrospective study. *Neurology.* 1992;42:801-8.

Penfield W. The cerebral cortex in man. I. The cerebral cortex and consciousness. *Arch Neurol Psychiatry.* 1938;40:417-42.

Penfield W. *The cerebral cortex of man.* Hafner, New York 1968.

Penfield W. *The excitable cortex in conscious man.* Liverpool University Press, Liverpool 1958.

Penfield W. The interpretive cortex: the stream of consciousness in the human brain can be electrically reactivated. *Science.* 1959;129:1719-25.

Penfield W. *The mystery of the mind: a critical study of consciousness and the human brain.* Princeton University Press, Princeton 1975.

Porter RJ. Disorders of consciousness and associated complex behaviors. *Semin Neurol.* 1991;11:110-7.

Prevett MC, Duncan JS, Jones T, Fish DR, Brooks DJ. Demonstration of thalamic activation during typical absence seizures using H2(15)O and PET. *Neurology.* 1995;45:1396-1402.

Rainville P, Hofbauer RK, Bushnell MC, Duncan GH, Price DD. Hypnosis modulates activity in brain structures involved in the regulation of consciousness. *J Cogn Neurosci.* 2002;14:887-901.

Reynders HJ, Broks P, Dickson JM, Lee CE, Turpin G. Investigation of social and emotion information processing in temporal lobe epilepsy with ictal fear. *Epilepsy Behav.* 2005;7:419-29.

Salek-Haddadi A, Lemieux L, Merschhemke M, Duncan JS, Fish DR. Imaging absence seizures using fMRI. *Epilepsia.* 2002;43(Suppl. 7):123.

Searle J. *The rediscovery of the mind.* MIT Press, Cambridge, MA 1992.

Shear J. *Explaining consciousness: the hard problem.* MIT Press, Cambridge, MA 1997.

Shin WC, Hong SB, Tae WS, Kim SE. Ictal hyperperfusion patterns according to the progression of temporal lobe seizures. *Neurology.* 2002;58:373-80.

Skokowski P. I, zombie. *Conscious Cogn.* 2002;11:1-9.

Snead OC. Basic mechanisms of generalised absence seizures. *Ann Neurol.* 1995;37:146-57.

Sno HN, Linszen DH. The déjà vu experience: remembrance of things past? *Am J Psychiatry.* 1990;1473:1587-95.

Spielberger CD, Gorsuch RL, Lushene RE. *Manual for the State-Trait Anxiety Inventory ("Self-evaluation Questionnaire").* Consulting Psychologists Press Inc, Palo Alto 1970.

Strauss E, Risser A, Jones MW. Fear responses in patients with epilepsy. *Arch Neurol.* 1982;39:626-30.

Taylor DC, Lochery M. Temporal lobe epilepsy: origin and significance of simple and complex auras. *J Neurol Neurosurg Psychiatry.* 1987;50:673-81.

Taylor DC, Marsh SM. Hughlings Jackson's Dr. Z: the paradigm of temporal lobe epilepsy revealed. *J Neurol Neurosurg Psychiatry.* 1980;43:758-67.

Taylor J, editor. *The selected writings of John Hughlings Jackson.* Basic Books, New York 1958.

Theodore WH, Porter RG, Penry JK. Complex partial seizures: clinical characteristics and differential diagnosis. *Neurology.* 1983;33:1115-21.

Van Paesschen W, Dupont P, Van Driel G, Van Billoen H, Maes A. SPECT perfusion changes during complex partial seizures in patients with hippocampal sclerosis. *Brain.* 2003;126:1103-11.

Van Paesschen W, King MD, Duncan JS, Connelly A. The amygdala and temporal lobe simple partial seizures: a prospective and quantitative MRI study. *Epilepsia.* 2001;42:857-62.

Vuilleumier P, Assal F, Blanke O, Jallon P. Distinct behavioral and EEG topographic correlates of loss of consciousness in absences. *Epilepsia.* 2000;41:687-93.

Weil AA. Ictal emotions occurring in temporal lobe dysfunction. *Arch Neurol.* 1959;1:86-97.

Weir B. The morphology of the spike-wave complex. *Electroencephalogr Clin Neurophysiol.* 1965;19:284-90.

Williams D. The structure of emotions reflecting in epilepsy experiences. *Brain.* 1956;79:29-67.

Yamauchi T. Impairment of consciousness during epileptic seizures with special reference to neuronal mechanisms. *Epilepsia.* 1998;39(Suppl 5):16-20.

Yeni SN, Kabasakal L, Yalcinkaya C, Nisli C, Dervent A. Ictal and interictal SPECT findings in childhood absence epilepsy. *Seizure.* 2000;9:265-9.

Zappulla RA. Epilepsy and consciousness. *Semin Neurol.* 1997;17:113-9.

Chapter 6

PROGRESSIVE LOSS OF CONSCIOUSNESS: ALZHEIMER'S DISEASE

Last scene of all,
that ends this strange eventful history,
is second childishness, and mere oblivion;
sans teeth, sans eyes, sans taste, sans everything.

W. Shakespeare, As you like it, Act II, Scene VII

6.1. WHEN CONSCIOUSNESS TURNS OFF

The loss of the ability to judge with increasing age was originally recognized and described by the Greeks Solon and Plato and the Roman Cicero (in *De Senectute*), albeit the term "*dementia*" was first introduced by the Roman physician Aulus Cornelius Celsus in his treatise *De Medicina* (20 AD), indicating in a generic way the alterations of intelligence and behaviour. However, until the XVIII century dementia was synonym of madness. In 1838 the French psychiatrist Jeanne-Etienne-Dominique Esquirol first defined dementia as a clinical picture characterized by loss of memory, ability to judge and attention, clearly distinguishing dementia, an acquired process, from congenital mental deficit (*"The oligophrenic is a poor, while the demented is a failure"*).

Alzheimer's disease (AD) is the most relevant cause of dementia among people aged 65 and over, and it raises the question of severe impairment of self-consciousness in an exemplary manner, as it involves disorders of memory as well as of other cognitive functions and leads to a progressive and inexorable mental and physical decay.

According to DSM-IV criteria (American Psychiatric Association 2000), the essential features of dementia include impairment in memory and at least another cognitive domain (language, visual-spatial skills, etc.), and significant disturbance of work or social functioning resulting from cognitive deficits. These features should not occur as isolated features of delirium. However, from a clinical point of view, the term "dementia" doesn't refer to a particular progressive and irreversible illness: it has to be considered a syndrome instead of a single disease. This syndrome includes cognitive symptoms (memory impairment, spatial and temporal disorientation, apraxia, aphasia, alexia, agraphia, abstract reasoning, acalculia, agnosia, visuo-spatial deficits) and non cognitive symptoms, such as delirium, hallucinations, affective disturbances (depression, euphoria, emotional lability), anxiety, neurovegetative symptoms (sleep, appetite, and sexual behaviour disorders), psychomotor activity disorders (vagabondage, afinalistic bustle, akathisia), agitation (physical and verbal aggressiveness, persistent vocalization), personality alterations (indifference, apathy, disinhibition, irritability).

The prevalence rate of dementia in the elderly (people over 65 years) is 5% (all causes) and it nearly doubles every subsequent five year, with a peak of 40% in subjects over 85. An almost exponential increase with age and a female preponderance have been described. The incidence rate also increases with age, but epidemiological data are limited (Woods et al. 2000).

The classical distinction between cortical dementia (with prevalent cortical lesions and early symbolic, abstract thinking and memory function alterations) and subcortical dementia (with neuropathological alteration in basal ganglia, thalamus, rostral brainstem and involvement of frontal lobe projections clinically characterized by early cognitive impairment, personality alterations with depression, apathy, inertia, motor slowdown) is no longer accepted because of the remarkable overlap of clinical manifestations and the impossibility of a precise neuroanatomical differentiation. It is worth remembering the frequent cognitive deficit in the elderly related to depressive syndromes rather than neurodegenerative disorders (so called "depressive pseudodementia"). It is not always easy to make a clear distinction between this clinical pattern and true dementia. Clinical features like a rapid and datable onset, a rapid progression of cognitive symptoms, and of course consciousness deficits, are useful for diagnosis. Most importantly, cognitive response to an anti-depressive therapy is suggestive of pseudodementia (Lee et al. 2003).

There exist several classifications of dementia; the most useful classification is the clinical one, that differentiates between primary and secondary dementias (Table 6.1)

The clinical syndrome of dementia may be caused by various diseases, each characterized by specific signs and symptoms constellation in combination with a specific underlying neuropathological substrate. Alzheimer's disease (AD) is the most common cause of dementia. It is a neurodegenerative disorder, generally assumed to be caused by neuritic plaques and neurofibrillary tangles which accumulate in the brain. The second common type of dementia is vascular dementia, which may be caused by a wide range of vascular pathologies affecting the brain, such as "large vessel" disease (large territorial or strategic infarctions) and "small vessel" disease (lacunes and white matter hyperintensities as seen in brain magnetic resonance imaging). Other frequent causes of degenerative dementia include frontotemporal lobar degeneration and dementia with Lewy bodies. From a clinical perspective, it is often difficult to reliably distinguish between these subtypes of dementia. The following section provides an overview on the different dementia syndromes.

Table 6.1. Etiologic classification of dementias

Primary (degenerative) dementias
Alzheimer's disease
Pick's disease
Not determined:
Primary progressive dysphasia
Dementia with Lewy bodies
Fronto-temporal dementia
Cortico-basal de generation
Secondary dementias
Vascular dementia
Prion disease dementia
Normal pressure hydrocephalus-associated dementia
Traumatic dementia (punch-drunk syndrome)
Cerebral neoplasia or extra cranial neoplasia-associated dementia
Endocrine-metabolic disease-associated dementia
Vitamin deficiency-associated dementia
Toxic and drug induced encephalopathy-associated dementia
Infectious disease-associated dementia

6.2. DEGENERATIVE DEMENTIAS

6.2.1. Alzheimer's Disease

Alzheimer's disease (or Alzheimer-Perusini's Disease) is a primary dementia first described by the German psychiatrist Alois Alzheimer in a seminal 1907 paper, and independently by the Italian scientist Gaetano Perusini in 1910. The "Alzheimer's disease" eponymous was suggested by Emil Kraepelin in the "Handbook of Psychiatry". It has been proposed to rename this condition with the double eponymous of Alzheimer-Perusini, thus acknowledging the two scientists who contributed to the identification of the syndrome. Augusta D. was the first patient described by Alzheimer (Figure 6.1). She was 51 when first showed a delusion with jealousy coupled with progressive memory deficit. After the patient's death at the age of 55 years, Alzheimer applied new staining techniques to the patient's brain tissue and demonstrated the presence of what is now termed neurofibrillary tangles and neuritic plaques in the neocortex and other brain regions.

For years, Alzheimer's disease (AD) was considered a presenile dementia, in part because some plaques and tangles occurred in elderly persons without dementia and some elderly persons with dementia had few plaques and tangles (Yaari and Corey-Bloom 2007). Such conflicts were resolved, however, in the late 1960s, when the degree of dementia was shown to correlate with the number of neuritic plaques in neocortical association areas. Moreover, causes of senile dementia other than AD were also recognized. There also exists familiar AD, associated with mutations of APP (amyloid protein precursor), PS (presenilin)-1, and PS-2.

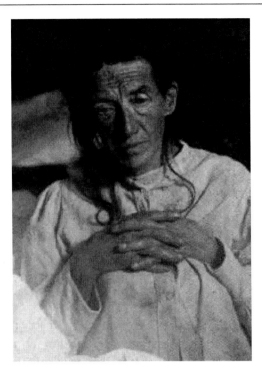

Figure 1. Augusta D, the first patient described by Dr Alzheimer (picture taken in 1902).

AD is the most common cause of dementia, accounting for approximately 50-60% of all cases. It is a degenerative disease with an insidious onset and an inexorable progression to the exitus in about ten years for infectious complications. Clinical features are as follow: AD does not exhibit a pattern of global decline from onset, but rather a relatively predictable one, including mainly three stages, with both cognitive and non cognitive symptoms. The most common presentation includes minimal temporal disorientation, word finding difficulties (with a relatively preserved comprehension), constructive apraxia (for three-dimensional drawings), complex problem solving impairment. Of note, in the early stages the patient exhibits preserved consciousness of his own progressive intellectual function impairment; anxiety, depression, thought disorders (like paranoid ideation) and personality disorders (apathy, irritability) are not uncommon. It is also possible an initial difficulty in daily life activities.

In the middle stages of the disease it is common to observe worsening of spatial and temporal disorientation, in particular failure of anterograde episodic memory, which interferes with daily life. Moreover, there is a severe complex problem solving deficit, language skills decline as the illness progresses with paraphasias, anomy, circumlocution, and comprehension deficits. Ideomotor apraxia also occurs, rendering tasks such as dressing and eating difficult. Insomnia, lack of appetite, bradykinesia and extrapyramidal signs are other typical manifestations of this stage. Patients need to be helped out for their personal care.

The late stages of AD are characterized by complete impairment of cognitive activities with remote memory loss for familiar faces and places. Language is seriously impaired up to mutism. There are also rigidity, bradykinesia, myoclonus, convulsive seizures; the patient can be aggressive, and often becomes incontinent. In the terminal phase he is no more able to communicate, is confined to bed and needs artificial feeding; sometimes he is in a vegetative state.

Etiology

Much research is being conducted looking for possible causes for Alzheimer's disease, which should lead to treatments that may delay or even halt the dementia process. Efforts have focused on various neurotransmitter systems, especially the cholinergic system, because of findings of loss of cholinergic neurons in the basal nucleus of the forebrain (Palmer et al. 1988).

AD risk factors are thoroughly investigated in order to find out the basic mechanisms leading to dementia. Age is a well known risk factor for dementia. In addition, female sex has repeatedly been shown to be associated with an increased risk of AD, especially at old age. Other risk factors for AD include vascular factors such as hypertension, diabetes mellitus, smoking, and heart disease (Casserly and Topol 2004). There are also some putative protective factors like the use of estrogens, non steroid anti-inflammatory drugs, and a high educational level.

AD is generally assumed to be caused by senile plaques made by amyloid, however it is not clear if these plaques are the cause rather than an epiphenomenon of the degeneration. Amyloid is cleaved from a larger transmembrane protein (β-amyloid precursor protein, APP) by the action of the enzymes β - and γ-secretases, and its formation is prevented by the action of α-secretase. In normal condition the α-secretase activity is prevalent, with the result of a slight amount of β-amyloid. In AD it seems to be prominent the β - and γ-secretases activity, leading to a major β-amyloid production. These deposits are widely distributed throughout the cerebral cortex and have a neurotoxic activity (Hardy and Selkoe 2002).

Some of the most recent discoveries have taken place in the area of molecular biology and genetics. The increased frequency of Down syndrome (trisomy 21) patients who invariably develop Alzheimer's disease neuropathology and dementia by their 40s elicited an initial focus on chromosome 21, and significant linkage to chromosome 21 was discovered in some early-onset families but not in others (Richards and Henry 1999). Only a small proportion of individuals with dementia suffer from a familiar form of dementia, caused by an autosomal dominant mutation. A few genetic loci have been identified through linkage studies. The APP gene (Amyloid precursor protein) is located on chromosome 21; whilst chromosome 14 hosts the presenilin 1 gene, that is responsible for 50% of the forms of early-onset familiar Alzheimer's disease. The presenilin 2 gene is located on chromosome 1 (Van der Flier and Scheltens 2005). Studies of the common late-onset disease (dementia beginning after age 60 years) showed evidence for linkage or association or both for a chromosome 19 region, which hosts the Apolipoprotein E (APOE) gene. APOE is involved in both lipid metabolism and cholesterol delivery. The APOE gene presents in three allelic forms (e2, e3, and e4). The e2 genotype has a protective effect, while risk of developing AD is higher for the e4 genotype. The e4/e4 genotype presents an earlier onset of the disease (Strittmatter and Roses 1995).

Neuropathology

Gross anatomy usually shows cerebral atrophy, which may be pronounced. In most cases, atrophy affects the whole cortex, but the occipital lobe may be relatively spared and the medial part of the temporal lobe (particularly the hippocampus) is generally more severely atrophic than other cortical areas. Occasionally the atrophy is predominantly frontal and temporal, and the appearance mimics that of the frontotemporal dementias (Boller et al. 1989). On microscopic examination, AD is characterized by a combination of abnormalities (Braak and Braak 1996):

- proteinaceous extracellular deposits: consist largely of a peptide known as β-amyloid. It is cleaved from a larger transmembrane protein (β-amyloid precursor protein) by the action of β - and γ-secretases, and its formation is prevented by the action of α-secretase. These deposits measure up to several hundreds micrometers in diameter and are widely distributed throughout the cerebral cortex. Plaques vary in appearance, and two main subtypes have been identified. Diffuse plaques consist largely of non-fibrillar extracellular β-amyloid. Neuritic plaques contain β-amyloid that is mostly in the form of amyloid fibrils, among which are irregularly swollen dystrophic neurites. The neurites are well visualized with silver stains. Microglia and astrocyte processes can be observed towards the periphery of neuritic plaques. Neuritic plaques may contain a dense central core of amyloid. Cerebral amyloid angiopathy (CAA) refers to the accumulation of β-amyloid in the walls of blood vessels (particularly arteries and arterioles) in the cerebral cortex and overlying leptomeninges and is an important cause of strokes in the elderly.

Cytoskeletal alterations are quite common. They are represented by neurofibrillary tangles - looped or twisted, skein-like aggregates of filamentous material, largely composed of hyperphosphorylated tau proteins. Most tangles are faintly basophilic. They can be impregnated with silver or immunostained for tau protein to facilitate their light microscopic detection. Tangles are located within the neuronal cell body and most often remain intraneuronal. However, when neurons degenerate, the tangles persist in the extracellular space, although they lose their basophilic properties and some of their affinity for silver salts. The swollen neurites that are present in neuritic plaques contain tangle-like material, and this also accumulates in fine nerve cell processes (known as neuropil threads) in proximity of the tangle bearing neurons.

Other abnormalities are represented by: 1) reduction in the density of synaptic proteins in the cerebral cortex; 2) neuronal loss, in particular loss of cholinergic neurons in the basal nucleus of the forebrain; 3) astrocytic gliosis; 4) microglial activation; 5) Hirano bodies (as in amyotrophic lateral sclerosis), eosinophilic rod structures located in dendrite of the hippocampus region; 6) vacuolar degeneration, i.e. cytoplasmatic vacuoles with an eosinophilic nucleus in the hippocampus pyramidal neurons.

Diagnosis

The definite diagnosis is possible only through the demonstration of typical macroscopic and microscopic lesions, at postmortem examination. *In vivo*, we can only estimate a probability of this disease with: clinical examination, laboratory tests (especially for the differential diagnosis of secondary dementia), neuropsychological tests and neuroradiology. Electroencephalography (EEG) shows diffuse slow activity (4-5 Hz), more evident with the disease progression. In the terminal stage, delta (1-2 Hz) activity may be present in the bilateral frontal regions.

- *Biomarkers:* Many biological markers have been proposed for the diagnosis of AD, but their real clinical utility remains uncertain (Knopman et al. 2001). Among the most studied ones, there are the cerebrospinal fluid levels of Tau protein and the soluble portion of APP; the metabolic properties of fibroblasts; the serum levels of melanotransferrin, and platelet APP forms (Growdon 1999; Padovani et al. 2002).

- *Clinical and functional neuroimaging studies:* A diagnostic evaluation for dementia includes a complete history (from a reliable informant); physical and neurological examination; neuropsychological examination; a few selected laboratory studies and neuroimaging. In this chapter we will only deal with the neuropsychological and neuroimaging investigations, because of their relevance for consciousness studies.

- *Neuropsychological examination:* Several tests may be employed for a complete neuropsychological evaluation of the demented patient (Cooper and Greene 2005; Kipps and Hodges 2005). One of the most commonly used in clinical practice for the assessment cognitive function is the *Mini-Mental State Examination (MMSE).* It provides useful information in grading established dementia, but does have limitations, particularly in detecting early dementia. The *Addenbrooke's cognitive assessment (ACE)* has been developed to overcome the shortcomings of the MMSE. Other tests, such as the *Short Test of Mental Status,* are specifically aimed at discriminating patients with dementia from normal subjects, whilst the *Blessed Information Memory Concentration Test* has been designed to evaluate the severity of dementia. The *Test for Severe Impairment* and the *Severe Impairment Battery* are used to follow the evolution of severely demented patients. Finally, a few other tests are employed to determine the impact of dementia on the social life and the functional autonomy of the patients. They are the *GMS-AGECAT Package,* including the *Geriatric Mental State Examination*, and the *Cambridge Examination for Mental Disorders of the Elderly (CAMDEX).* For the functional diagnosis the most commonly employed tools are the *ADL (Activity Daily Living)* and the *Instrumental Activity Daily Living (IADL).* The *Clinical Assessment of Psychopathology among the Elderly Residents (CAPER)* and the *Neuropsychiatric Inventory-UCLA-NPI* are used in the objective evaluation of behavioural disturbances in demented patients, while the *Cornell Scale for Depression in Dementia* and the *NIMH-Dementia Mood Assessment Scale* are used more specifically for mood disorder comorbidity.

- *Neuroradiological examination:* The main clinical application of neuroimaging is the differential diagnosis between the structural and physiological modifications of normal brain ageing and the several pathological conditions associated to dementia. A brain computer tomographic (CT) scan is usually *per se* sufficient to diagnose AD and rule out other neurological disorders, such as cerebrovascular disease, normal pressure hydrocephalus, subdural haematoma or brain tumor. Magnetic resonance imaging (MRI) can show small subcortical lacunae and mesial temporal lobe atrophy (Knopman et al. 2001). Single proton emission computer tomography (SPECT) may be helpful in atypical, difficult or early cases of AD (Richards and Hendrie 1999; Talbot et al. 1998).

In AD there is a characteristic hypoperfusion in the temporal and parietal lobes. In cerebrovascular disease there are more patchy changes, whilst Pick's disease is characterized by frontal and temporal lobes perfusion deficits. Positron emission tomography (PET) is employed for research purposes (especially for cognitive neuropsychological testing), but has limited clinical applications . Finally, functional MRI (fMRI) is commonly employed to evaluate the functional modifications of brain networks in AD or vascular dementia (Iacoboni et al. 1999).

The clinical diagnostic criteria for AD have been established by NINCDS (National Institute of Neurological Communicative Disorders and Stroke) (McKhann et al. 1984):

- Possible Alzheimer: dementia syndrome without impairment of consciousness in the absence of other known causes.
- Probable Alzheimer: dementia syndrome confirmed by clinical observation and neuropsychological tests following the exclusion of a secondary dementia.
- Definite Alzheimer: the same clinical criteria plus microscopic diagnosis.

The most reliable diagnostic procedure is the association between TC and SPECT in Possible and Probable AD categories. An insidious onset, the presence of neurological focal signs, convulsions and deambulation impairment in the early stages are suggestive of a misdiagnosed AD.

6.2.2. Pick's Disease

This kind of dementia was first described by Arnold Pick at the end of the XIX century and accounts for 1% of all cases (Kertesz 2006). It frequently has a genetic origin (autosomal dominant transmission) and a presenile onset, leading to death in 2-10 years. The clinical distinction from AD is often impossible. In Pick's disease behavioral impairment and loss of judgment ability seems to prevail, whereas spatial orientation is usually preserved. Primitive reflexes and extrapyramidal signs are frequently observed. Neuroradiological exams show a fronto-temporal atrophy; whilst the neuropathological pattern is characterized by marked fronto-temporal cortical atrophy, usually asymmetric and with a relative conservation of the superior temporal circumvolution. Pick bodies are intraneuronal inclusions made by stored helix filaments. In a few atypical cases, there are no Pick bodies, whereas there are swelling neurons with stored intermediate filaments with ubiquitin. Investigators still ignore if this condition should be considered an independent form of dementia rather than a subtype of fronto-temporal dementia (Kertesz 2006).

6.2.3. Frontotemporal Dementia

Frontotemporal degeneration is associated with a focal and often asymmetric degeneration of the frontal and temporal lobes, accounting for approximately 10-15% of all cases of dementia (Neary et al. 1998; Johnson et al. 2005). The etiology of this condition is unknown. The initial presentation may be subtle but is characterized by personality changes, emotional disturbances, and behavioral problems. Patients may appear apathetic, socially withdrawn, inappropriately jocular, disinhibited, facetious, or unmotivated. In the clinical evolution we can highlight temporal (Kluver-Bucy like syndrome) and extrapyramidal signs. The onset is usually among the fifth and the seventh decade of life. Forty percent of cases, especially the earlier onset ones, seem to have genetic origin, with a possible association with tau protein mutation on chromosome 17.

The neuropathological changes seen in FTD are not specific (McKhann et al. 2001). In 20% of FTD it is possible to find Pick bodies. Many cases are associated with tau inclusions, but mild spongiform changes with neuronal loss and gliosis may occur in the absence of inclusions. The clinical phenotype reflects the anatomical distribution of the pathology, rather than the particular pathological process. The differential diagnosis with AD is difficult: both these patient groups meet NINCDS criteria. It is possible to distinguish the two forms of dementia by clinical, neuropsychological and neuroradiological data.

Primary progressive dysphasia (Amici et al. 2006) is a progressive decline in language output that occurs with a relative absence of other psychological deficits. Speech is non-fluent, effortful, and lacking in prosody. Articulation is disturbed, word-finding pauses occur, and syntactic errors are prominent. The communication difficulties are evident to both the patient and the observer. Repetition and reading aloud are impaired, and there is pronounced anomia. Patients have difficulties reciting the days of the week or similar well rehearsed series. With disease progression speech becomes unintelligible. Comprehension is, by contrast, relatively preserved. Neuroradiological examinations show a perisilvian atrophy of the dominant hemisphere. This kind of dementia has a presenile onset, a low prevalence and a high familiarity. The pathogenesis is unknown.

A distinctive form is the so called semantic dementia, in which patients display increasingly empty, circumlocutory speech, reflecting the profound loss of semantic knowledge (Knibb and Hodges 2005). Presenting complaints may relate to forgetting the names of things with unawareness of the parallel decline in word comprehension. The fluent dysphasia observed in such patients is characteristically coupled with severe anomia and reduced vocabulary.

6.2.4. Movement Disorders Associated With Dementia

Extrapyramidal signs are detected in 30-60% of cases of dementia. Conversely, 20-30% of patients with Parkinson's disease have a frank dementia pattern and 30-40% have a cognitive impairment. The clinical picture resembles a "prefrontal" deafferentiation state (attention impairment, memory recall deficit, executive dysfunctions). A few different clinical patterns have been described:

- Parkinson's dementia: Parkinson's disease responsive to L-Dopa that ultimately causes dementia.
- Dementia with Lewy bodies (DLB): dementia, parkinsonism, and hallucinations-like symptoms.
- AD with extrapyramidal sings: AD patients that develop parkinsonian signs.

We will now focus on DLB and corticobasal degeneration (CBD), because of the peculiar alterations in conscious perception which characterize these conditions.

Dementia with Lewy Bodies (DLB)

Lewy bodies are neuronal concentric, cytoplasmatic and ialine inclusions composed of abnormally phosphorylated neurofilament proteins aggregated with ubiquitin, that are deposited in brainstem nuclei, paralimbic, and neocortical areas. The clinical phenotype of patients with DLB involves visual hallucinations, parkinsonism, and fluctuating attention and alertness with intervals of lucidity (McKeith et al. 1996). The visual hallucinations are typically well formed and detailed. Hallucinations occur in other modalities not uncommonly and delusions also are a feature. The cognitive profile reflects a combination of cortical and subcortical disease. There is cognitive slowing with impairment of frontal executive functions and attention. In addition, there are pronounced visuospatial and memory problems implicating parieto-occipital regions. The presence of aphasia, agnosia, and apraxia may lead to a misdiagnosis of AD. Along with the cognitive effects, DLB is associated with repeated falls and episodes of transient loss of consciousness. There are also REM phase sleep disorders. Sleep studies are useful and show a generalized muscular atony during REM phase. Clonazepam is indicated in these sleep disorders. Cognitive impairments may develop before or after parkinsonism symptoms and signs including akinesia, rigidity, and tremor.

There are two different pathological patterns: 1) pure DLB, and 2) AD with cortical Lewy bodies. Lewy bodies are also present in 80% of patients of Parkinson's disease, even if dementia in these cases follows the akinetic-hypertonic syndrome. The differential diagnosis should be posed with other conditions that are responsible of parkinsonism-associated dementia, such as neuroleptic use and AD with extrapyramidal signs.

Corticobasal Degeneration

Corticobasal degeneration (CBD) usually presents with an asymmetric akinetic-rigid syndrome, progressing to death within 4-6 years (Mahapatra et al. 2004). Ideomotor limb apraxia is often observed and there are associated visuospatial and constructional difficulties. The *alien hand* sign (spontaneous, coordinated hand movements outside of the patient's control) may develop in one limb. This may be associated with cortical sensory loss, dysarthria, ataxia, chorea, pyramidal signs, dysarthria and/or orofacial apraxia. Dyscalculia and nonfluent aphasia may be observed and frontal dysfunction may also occur. Memory impairment is typically less pronounced than that observed in AD. Despite the presence of these neuropsychological symptoms at the presentation of the disease, CBD is usually classified among the movement disorders.

6.3. VASCULAR DEMENTIA

Vascular dementia accounts for 15% of all cases of dementia. The prevalence is higher according to aging and in subjects over 85 years is similar to the prevalence of AD. The incidence is about 1%. Risk factors include: a previous stroke, risk factors for stroke (hypertension, heart disease, smoke, high cholesterol levels, diabetes), low educational level, high alcohol consumption, and cerebral atrophy. The clinical picture in vascular dementia depends on the location, size, and number of the infarcts. The diagnosis relies on the clinical picture, brain imaging findings and the presence of predisposing factors (Roman et al. 1993). There is commonly an accumulation of neurological and neuropsychological deficits. There may be multiple cortical infarcts causing a ''step-wise'' deterioration in function. Dysarthria, dysphagia, rigidity, visuospatial deficits, ataxia, and pyramidal or extrapyramidal signs may occur, depending on the site of the pathology. Alternatively, subcortical deficits may occur exclusively, with infarcts involving the thalamus, basal ganglia, or internal capsule. These may present without any sudden deteriorations, rather manifesting as impaired attention and poor executive function. It is important to differentiate this syndrome from other causes of subcortical dementia and it may coexist with other dementias – e.g., AD (Langa et al. 2004).

The term ''vascular dementia'' is hampered by lack of agreement regarding definition. It comprises several different entities:

- multi-infarct dementia (MID): recurrent transient ischemic attacks (TIAs) or strokes followed in a short period of time by dementia. There are often cortical infarcts caused by thromboembolisms of main arteries.
- strategic single infarct dementia: thalamus, angular gyrus, bilateral hippocampus.
- diffuse small vessel ischemia: chronic ischemic state of the white sub-cortical matter.
- chronic hypoperfusion state.

Other types of vascular dementia include (Aggarwal and Decarli 2007):

- *Binswanger's disease*: pattern of disease characterized by multiple ischemic lacunar lesions (basal ganglia, thalamus, pons) associated with hemispheric white matter ischemic demyelization and a syndrome of cognitive impairment, focal neurological deficits, gait apraxia, pseudobulbar palsy, and urinary incontinence. Urinary and gait disturbances typically occur relatively early in the disease course and sometimes precede overt signs of cognitive impairment.
- *Thalamic dementia*: disease characterised by bilateral lacunar lesions in the anterior paramedian thalamus, which cause a fronto-limbic syndrome with apathy, amnesia, and psycho-motor impairment.
- *Cerebral autosomal dominant arteriopathy with subcortical infarcts and leucoencephalopathy (CADASIL)* is a rare familiar vascular dementia with a typical onset most in the fourth decade, with recurrent transient ischaemic attacks (TIAs) or strokes. Migraine, generally with aura, develops in half of cases, usually a few years before the first vascular events. Neurological symptoms may be preceded by psychiatric manifestations, most commonly depression, in a substantial minority.

Epilepsy can occur, but is uncommon. The disease progresses initially with recurrent vascular events with recovery, but as disability increases these discrete events tend to merge and the condition becomes gradually progressive.

It is caused by mutation of the notch 3 gene, which codes for a large transmembrane receptor. The gene is expressed in vascular smooth muscle cells in a variety of organs and mutated genes cause accumulation of the extracellular portion of the receptor within blood vessel walls. This material was originally noted to be PAS positive on light microscopy, and on electron microscopy is seen as a granular osmiophilic deposit (GOM) within vessel walls adjacent to smooth muscle cells. These changes may be seen in a variety of tissues but it is in the brain that the pathology gives rise to clinically apparent disease.

6.4. OTHER DEMENTIA SYNDROMES

6.4.1. Normal Pressure Hydrocephalus

First described by Hakim and Adams a few decades ago (Hakim and Adams 1965), the clinical syndrome of symptomatic hydrocephalus with normal cerebrospinal fluid pressure should be suspected if the clinical triad of gait apraxia, subcortical dementia, and urinary dysfunction are present (so-called *Hakim and Adams triad*). It is a silent communicating hydrocephalus that evolves without the classical symptoms of elevated intracranial pressure. The feet are said to show the "glued to the floor" sign when the patient tries to walk. Imaging shows ventricular dilatation out of proportion to the degree of sulcal enlargement.

Overall, this is a rare disease, with an onset in the sixth decade, accounting for 1-5% of all dementia case; it can be idiopathic or linked to cerebral lesions like meningoencephalitis or subarachnoideal hemorrhage. The currently accepted denomination is *adult chronic hydrocephalus,* because of the demonstration of transient rise of cerebrospinal fluid pressure, mainly during sleep (Bret et al. 2002). In selected cases, treatment is neurosurgical and consists of ventricular-peritoneal derivation.

6.4.2. Traumatic Dementia

This progressive chronic encephalopathy is the manifestation of the brain injury caused by repeated minor traumas (*punch-drunk syndrome*), characteristic of boxers (Starkstein and Jorge 2005). It is clinically characterized by progressive mental impairment with memory loss, ideo-motor slowdown, loss of critical ability, irritability and aggressiveness. It is frequently associated to a Parkinsonian syndrome.

6.5. MILD COGNITIVE IMPAIRMENT

Patients with profound memory loss without other cognitive impairment and patients with minor impairments in different cognitive domains but no functional impairment at work or home do not meet the criteria for dementia and are currently classified as having the so-called *mild cognitive impairment (MCI)*, a clinical condition previously defined *benign forgetfulness senescence* (Kral 1962). It has been hypothesized that patients evolving to frank dementia may reach an intermediate stage characterized by the dysfunction of a single cognitive domain, which in most cases is memory (Petersen et al. 1999). The diagnosis is based on the following criteria (Petersen 2004): 1) report (by the patient or an informant) of memory loss; 2) abnormal memory performance for age and scholarity; 3) normal general cognition; 4) normal activities of daily living; 5) criteria for dementia not met. Longitudinal studies have shown that as many as 15% of such patients may develop dementia, usually of Alzheimer's type (Ritchie and Touchon 2000).

RM studies have shown that hippocampal atrophy, observed in AD and FTD patients, is a typical feature of MCI patients too, and seems to be a potential predictive index of its evolution to dementia, although it is not known if the final phenotype will be AD or FTD (Blass et al. 2004).

6.6. THE MANAGEMENT OF DEMENTIA

Early diagnosis of AD is essential (Kawas 2003), as it allows patients, caregivers and doctors to adopt strategies to possibly slow the cognitive decline, and gives them time to plan for the future. The management of definite AD involves multiple modalities (pharmacological, psychological and social); furthermore, the legal aspects of assisting patients with progressive loss of consciousness are not secondary.

The pharmacological management aims to treat the cognitive impairment and the consequent behavioural disturbances (Mayeaux and Sano 1999) . As AD is characterized by degeneration of basal forebrain cholinergic systems, one strategy for improving AD symptoms is to enhance cholinergic neurotransmission.

Inhibitors of the acetylcholinesterase enzyme (tacrine, donepezil, rivastagmine, galantamine) enhance cholinergic neurotransmission and are therefore considered a standard therapy for AD patients (Doody et al. 2001; Cummings 2004). Tacrine, a first-generation acetylcholinesterase inhibitor, is now rarely used, because of its hepatotoxicity. All cholinesterase inhibitors provide symptomatic relief without altering the course of the disease. A new promising agent s metrifonate, a pro-drug for the long-acting cholinesterase inhibitor 2,2-dichlorovinyl-dimethylphosphate.

Memantine, an N-methyl-D-Aspartate antagonist, is thought to interfere with glutamatergic excitoxicity pathways, and may provide symptomatic improvement by exerting positive effects on the function of hippocampal neurons (Parsons et al. 1999).

No antiamyloid therapies are currently available. A program to vaccinate humans was implemented after the observation that immunization with beta-amyloid reduces AD pathological signs in transgenic mice that have the APP mutation (Schenk et al. 1999), but the clinical trial was interrupted as encephalitis developed in 6% of patients (Orgogozo et al. 2003). Vitamin E as an antioxidant agent is employed at high doses by many practitioners, but significant data on its effectiveness are lacking. The same can be said for other neuroprotective strategies targeting lipid peroxidation at the level of cell membranes, inflammation, and hyperphosphorilation of tau protein. Several other agents (including herbal supplements and the so-called nutraceuticals) are usually employed on empirical basis in clinical practice as putative preventive strategies.

The management of the *Behavioural and Psychological Symptoms of Dementia (BPSD)* – i.e. personality changes, mood disorders, and psychotic disturbances associated to cognitive impairment in demented subjects - is both pharmacological and psychosocial (Reisberg et al 1987; Assal and Cummings 2002). Atypical antipsychotic agents (risperidone, olanzapine, quetiapine, ziprasidone and aripiprazole) are the preferred medications for the management of psychosis or agitation. Mood-stabilizing agents (carbamazepine or valproic acid) may reduce behavioural disturbances, and selective serotonin reuptake inhibitors (SSRI) (e.g. citalopram, paroxetine, sertraline, fluoxetine), noradrenergic reuptake inhibtors (e.g. mirtazapine) and mixed noradrenergic-serotoninergic reuptake inhibitors (e.g. venlafaxine) are commonly used in the treatment of depression in AD patients (Cummings 2004). Benzodiazepines must be used with caution, as they may cause significant behavioural and cognitive side effects (Stern et al. 1991).

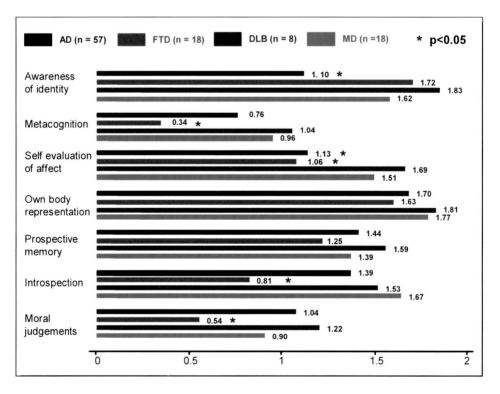

Figure 2. Comparison of self–reflection dimensions in four dementia groups (SCQ subscales, mean scores).

6.7. REFLECTIVE CONSCIOUSNESS IN PATIENTS WITH DEMENTIA

A recent study by the authors of this volume investigated reflective consciousness in a population of patients with degenerative dementias, with special attention to the relationship between alteration of RC and the natural history/neuropsychiatric profile of the disease. A total of 103 outpatients attending the Dementia Clinic were recruited. Inclusion criteria were (1) diagnosis of mild or moderate degenerative dementia according to DSM-IV and NINCDS/ADRDA criteria, and (2) age-corrected Mini-Mental State Examination (MMSE) >10. All patients underwent a comprehensive neuropsychological examination and neuropsychiatric assessment for behavioural and psychological signs and symptoms of dementia (BPSD). RC was indexed in each subject using a specifically developed 14-item Self-Consciousness Questionnaire (SCQ) (Gil et al. 2001). Four groups of patients were studied: 57 patients with Alzheimer's disease (AD); 18 with frontotemporal dementia (FTD); 8 with dementia with Lewy bodies (DLB); 18 with mixed dementia (MD). The four groups did not differ in terms of clinical severity (CDR scores) and cognitive dysfunction (MMSE scores). However, patients with FTD scored significantly lower than other dementia groups on the SCQ (especially questions on moral judgement, introspection, metacognition, and self evaluation of the affective state), whilst patients with AD showed marked deficits in awareness of identity and self evaluation of affect (Figure 6.2).

Moreover, total SCQ scores correlated significantly with the frontal function tests - Frontal Assessment Battery, FAB; Middelheim Frontality Score, MFS - but did not show any correlation with other clinical characteristics including BPSD ratings, as assessed with the Neuropsychiatric Inventory (NPI) and the Cornell Scale for Depression in Dementia (CSDD). These results suggest that reflective consciousness is a multifaceted concept, which is more severely affected in patients with FTD than in patients with other forms of degenerative dementia, regardless of the degree of cognitive deficit. With respect to RC domains, FTD seems to be characterised by selective deficit in moral and self judgements, as predicted by predominant involvement of the frontal lobe; on the other hand, patients with AD show a predominant impairment in awareness of identity and self evaluation of affect, consistent with the early involvement of posteromedial parietal regions involved in the "default mode of brain function", and subserving self processing and first-person perspective (Cavanna and Trimble 2006; Greicius et al. 2004).

6.8. THE NEUROBIOLOGY OF THE DWINDLING SELF

The concept of "self" has been the main subject of reflection for literates, philosophers, psychologists, and scientists for centuries, as it stands as the central nucleus in the theoretical consideration of the uniqueness of human beings. To be able to "reflect" on his own self allows man to ask the fundamental questions about life and death, and eventually to give meaning to human events.

The lexical definitions of "self" (*se* in Latin) are quite unsatisfactory: most dictionaries use terms that refer to the essential qualities of a person, i.e. the ones that distinguish one individual from another. As "se" is the accusative form of the nominative pronoun "I" (*ego* in Latin), it can be implicitly considered as the ego observed by itself. In other words, with a philosophical expression, we might say that the *se, per se,* is synonymous with self reflection or, in a more extensive view, with self (or auto)consciousness (*autòs* is the Greek term for self). However, this hermeneutical (interpretative) loop is autoreferential and hence limitative, as it does not provide any insight into the mechanisms of either creation or development of the self within the complex architecture of consciousness. In this sense, the famous aphorism of Descartes *"Cogito ergo sum" (I think, therefore I am),* although illuminating in its geniality, is only partially true, as it clearly identifies consciousness with thinking, and thinking with living, but does not specify the main object of thinking (i.e., of the reflection), which is the self. The *ego* and the *se* are the subject (nominative) and the object (accusative) of the constitutive and founding dyad of consciousness, and allegorically stand one in front of the other, observing themselves reciprocally, in a mirror-fashioned (self- or autoreflecting) manner.

Due to the enormous progresses in scientific research in the last decades, also the concept of self has become feasible to neurobiological investigation (Miller et al. 2001). In particular, evidence in this field is derived from patients with AD or other types of dementia, as these disorders, as stated at the beginning of this chapter, raise the fundamental question of impairment of self-consciousness (Gil et al. 2001). AD involves alterations of memory, and memory is intimately linked to self-consciousness, since the awareness of one's own history is one of the multiple aspects of the so-called self-awareness, which includes, among the others, awareness of the body and awareness of perceptions (Zeman et al. 1997).

Clinical studies of self-consciousness in AD patients have mainly concerned the investigation of anosognosia, i.e. the lack of awareness of their condition or "loss of insight" (Ott et al. 1996). Anosognosia is used interchangeably to describe the impaired judgement of AD subjects concerning their own cognition, mood, behavior, or daily activities (Vasterling et al. 1995). It is related to the degree of cognitive deficits and involvement of frontal function (Migliorelli et al. 1995; Starkstein et al. 1996; Lopez and Becker 1993). A degree of anosognosia for cognitive impairment seems intrinsic in AD patients, and this would also explain the trend towards higher levels of anosognosia with greater severity of dementia (Zanetti et al. 1999). A score discrepancy between patient's and caregiver's assessments of cognitive function is one of the most frequently used measures of anosognosia, and a high discrepancy has been related to impaired activity in the superior frontal sulcus and the parietal cortex of AD subjects (Salmon et al. 2005). According to some authors, anosognosia for cognitive deficits in AD could be partly explained by impaired metabolism in the networks subserving self-referential processes (e.g., the superior frontal sulcus) and perspective-taking tasks (e.g., the temporoparietal junction). Interestingly, it has been hypothesized that AD patients are severely impaired in seeing themselves from a third-person perspective, i.e. to see themselves as other people see them. This ability would correspond to the "observing self", as defined by Baars et al. (2003). It is tempting to make a parallelism with the mirror-fashioned manner of conceptualizing consciousness, as if the mind of a patient suffering from AD would be forced (locked) into an autoreferential condition of self-

or autoconsciousness, with a progressive inability to get out of the vicious circle of self-reflection, and to assume the role of the self which observes without being observed (i.e., in a condition of free thinking and will). Thus, paradoxically, the study of progressive loss of consciousness in AD might represent a neuroscientific challenge to the neurobiological investigation of the millenary conundrum of free will and, consequently, moral responsibility (Roskies 2006).

The concept of "will", i.e. the motivation to maintain self-schemas derived from past social experience, is one of the three crucial cognitive domains of the self, the others being autobiographical and semantic memory (Greenwald and Pratkanis 1984). The latter is influenced by educational processes, starting with the perceptive knowledge of the physical world (including language) and the environment. Both autobiographical memory and motivation share neuroanatomical correlates in the frontal lobes (Stuss and Benson 1986), and maturation of the self develops with myelination of frontal structures (Sowell et al. 1999).

FTD has long been known to affect anterior frontal and temporal areas, and recent studies performed in FTD patients showed an involvement of the right hemisphere and the frontal lobes (Miller et al. 2001), suggesting that asymmetry itself would be a factor in the loss of self, beyond frontal function deficits. In other words, it would seem that a non dominant frontal lobe process, connecting the individual *ego* to both his previous relevant emotional experiences (i.e., autobiographical memory) and his own memories underlying self-schemas (i.e., will), is the neurobiological mechanism responsible for holding together the self. The loss of these two domains of the self would render the self vulnerable to change. Therefore, it has been proposed that normal nondominant frontal lobe function is essential for the maintenance of the integrity of the self.

Another recent study in patients with FTD, aimed at evaluating the emotional and somatic responses to a loud, sudden, and unexpected startle stimulus. This research demonstrated profound differences in the emotional self-conscious response (i.e. embarrassment) with respect to cognitively normal controls (Sturm et al. 2006). The authors suggest that this reduction in the degree of self-consciousness in FTD correlates with the neuronal loss in the medial prefrontal cortex. Indirect support for this speculation derives from other findings concerning self-conscious emotional behaviour in patients with selective injury to the orbitofrontal cortex, who, in contrast to FTD patients, express heightened self-conscious emotions (Beer et al. 2003). These patients typically present with intact anterior cingulated and anterior insula cortices, and thus, in keeping with the model proposed in FTD patients, should be able to produce self-conscious emotions. However, since consciousness requires the synthesis of information from neural networks located in different brain areas and involved in the processing of sensory data, memory and emotions (Delacour 1995), lesions in other structures, such as the ones observed in the hippocampus both in AD and FTD patients (Blass et al. 2004), could also explain impairment of conscious retrieval of information (Squire 1992). Finally, the disconnection of the dorsolateral prefrontal cortex hypothesized for AD could account for the difficulties/impairment in the sequential organization of information (Benson 1994), while the disconnection of the rostral-most part of the frontal lobe could account for difficulties in ensuring synthesis. This might be responsible for the difficulty of "concentrating attention on life", which seems to be the common denominator of self-consciousness alterations in AD patients (Gil et al. 2001).

Moreover, AD is by far the most common cause of bilateral pathological involvement in the medial surface of the parietal lobes, a brain region that has recently received particular attention for its pivotal role in self-consciousness and self-reflection. Although it has been known for some time that regional decreases in cerebral blood flow exist in both aging and dementia, more recent imaging studies have shown that the hypometabolism in AD is localized to specific cortical regions, including the precuneus and posterior cingulate (Minoshima et al. 1997; Buckner et al. 2000; Scahill et al. 2002; Good 2003; Lustig et al. 2003; Greicius et al. 2004).

These results accord well with findings of early neuropathological studies. Moreover, Reiman et al. (1996) demonstrated that subjects homozygous for the e4 allele for APOE, who are at higher risk of developing AD, display reduced rates of glucose metabolism in the posterior medial and lateral parietal cortices. A selective vulnerability of the posteromedial parietal cortex, including the precuneus, has also been noted in acute hypoxia due to carbon monoxide poisoning (Laureys et al. 1999), and has been ascribed to its unique arterial blood supply, positioned at the terminal branches of the anterior, middle, and posterior cerebral arteries. This arterial arrangement, which has no other counterpart in the cerebral cortex, may render the precuneus and surrounding areas particularly vulnerable to vascular diseases that affect the elderly. Raichle et al. (2001) wondered whether the exceptionally high metabolic rate exhibited by the precuneus and posterior cingulate adds to their vulnerability.

Recent MRI studies have found additional evidence suggesting that patterns of resting-state connectivity are decreased in normal aging but more so in patients having dementia (Lustig et al. 2003; Greicius et al. 2004). Thus, departures from a normal degree of default-mode activity may be important in the clinical etiology of age-related brain diseases (Van Horn 2004). Furthermore, the observed deactivations of the precuneus and posteromedial cortex when involved in goal-oriented behaviours (TIDs) show peculiar changes in populations with AD and mild cognitive impairment. In fact, AD patients fail to deactivate from the hypermetabolic activity of the resting state, and instead display a pattern of moderate precuneus activation with the onset of a cognitive task. Lustig et al. (2003) proposed that this slight activation may be the result of damage of the major projection pathways from the entorhinal cortex to the posterior cingulate and medial parietal cortices, given that pathological damage to the entorhinal cortex is a hallmark of AD. However, given the commonality of projections from the anterior intralaminar nuclei of the thalamus to all regions of the medial parietal cortex, Parvizi et al. (2006) suggest that such connections are central to the function of the precuneus and interrelated medial parietal areas at rest and during goal-directed tasks. Therefore the progressive damage to the thalamocortical pathways observed during ageing and AD may contribute to the observed reversal of deactivation patterns in elderly and demented populations. The finding that the anterior intralaminar nuclei of the thalamus are progressively affected by AD-related cytoscheletal pathology (Rub et al. 2002) strengthens this hypothesis. Some behavioural features of AD, including loss of arousal and self-awareness, could all be partially accounted for by the abnormal neuropathological changes affecting the functional connectivity between the anterior intralaminar nuclei and the precuneus. Our understanding of the neural correlates of the progressive deterioration of self-awareness and higher-order self-reflection is still at its very beginning: it is plausible that the combined use of rigorous clinical assessment measures and sophisticated brain imaging techniques will shed more light on the multiple neural mechanisms involved.

6.9. REFERENCES

Aggarwal NT, Decarli C. Vascular dementia: emerging trends. *Semin Neurol.* 2007;27:66-77.

American Psychiatric Association. DSM-IV-tr: diagnostic and statistical manual of mental disorders. 4th edn, text revision. Washington, DC: American Psychiatric Association, 2000.

Amici S, Gorno-Tempini ML, Ogar JM, Dronkers NF, Miller BL. An overview on primari progressive aplasia and its variants. *Behav Neurol* 2006;17:77-87.

Assal F, Cummings JL. Neuropsychiatric symptoms in the dementias. *Current Opin Neurol.* 2002;15;445-50.

Baars BJ, Ramsoy TZ, Laureys S. Brain, conscious experience and the observing self. *Trends Neurosci.* 2003;26:671-5

Beer JS, Heerey EA, Keltner D, Scabini D, Knight RT. The regulatory function of self-conscious emotion: insights from patients with orbitofrontal damage. *J Pers Soc Psychol.* 2003;85:594-604

Blass DM, Hatampaa KJ, Brandt J, Rao V, Steinberg M, Troncoso JC, Rabins PV. Dementia in hippocampal sclerosis resembles frontotemporal dementia more than Alzheimer disease. *Neurology.* 2004;63:492-7

Boller F, Lopez OL, Moosy J. Diagnosis of dementia: clinicalpathologic correlations. *Neurology.* 1989;39:76-9

Braak H, Braak E. Evolution of the neuropathology of Alzheimer's disease. *Acta Neurol Scand.* 1996;165:3-12

Bret P, Guyotat J, Chazal J. Is normal pressure hydrocephalus a valid concecpt in 2002? A reappraisal in five questions and proposal for a new designation of the syndrome as "chronic hydrocephalus". *J Neurol Neurosurg Psychiatry.* 2002;73:9-12

Buckner RL, Snyder AZ, Sanders AL, Raichle ME, Morris JC. Functional brain imaging of young, nondemented, and demented older adults. *J Cogn Neurosci.* 2000;12(Suppl 2):24-34.

Casserly I, Topol E. Convergence of atherosclerosis and Alzheimer's disease: inflammation, cholesterol, and misfolded proteins. *Lancet.* 2004;363:1139-46

Cavanna AE, Trimble MR. The precuneus: a review of its functional anatomy and behavioral correlates. *Brain.* 2006;129:564-83.

Cooper S, Greene JDW. The clinical assessment of the patient with early dementia. *J Neurol Neurosurg Psychiatry.* 2005;76(suppl 5):15-24

Cummings JL. Alzheimers's disease. *N Engl J Med.* 2004;351:56-67

Delacour J. An introduction to the biology of consciousness. *Neuropsychologia.* 1995;33:1061-74

Doody RS, Stevens JC, Beck C. Dubinsky RM, Kaye JA, Gwyther L, Mohs RC, Thal LJ, Whitehouse PJ, DeKosky ST, Cummings JL. Practice parameters: management of dementia (an evidence based review): report of the Quality Standards Subcommittee of the American Academy of Neurology. *Neurology.* 2001;56:1154-66

Friedland RP, Wilcock GK. *Dementia.* In Evans JG. et al (eds), Oxford Textbook of Geriatric Medicine, Oxford University Press, Oxford 2000:922-31

Gil R, Arroyo-Anllo EM, Ingrand P, Gil M, Neau JP, Ornon C, Bonnaud V. Self-consciouness and Alzheimer's disease. *Acta Neurol Scand.* 2001;104:296-300

Good CD. Dementia and ageing: imaging in clinical neuroscience. *Br Med Bull.* 2003;65:159-68.

Greenwald AG, Pratkanis AR. *The self.* Erlbaum: Hillsdale, NJ 1984

Greicius MD, Srivastava G, Reiss AL, Menon V. Default-mode network activity distinguishes Alzheimer's disease from healthy aging: evidence from functional MRI. *Proc Natl Acad Sci.* 2004;101:4637-42.

Growdon JH. Biomarkers of Alzheimer disease. *Arch Neurol.* 1999;56:281-3

Hakim S, Adams RD. The special clinical problem of symptomatic hydrocephalus with normal cerebrospinal fluid hydrodynamics. *J Neurol Sci.* 1965;2:307-27

Hardy J, Selkoe DJ. The amyloid hypothesis of Alzheimer's disease: progress and problems on the road to therapeutics. *Science.* 2002;297:2209

Iacoboni M, Baron JC, Frackowiak RS, Mazziotta JC, Lenzi GL. Emission tomography contribution to clinical neurology. *Clin Neurophysiol.* 1999;110:2-23

Johnson JK, Diehl J, Mendez MF, Neuhaus J, Shapira JS, Forman M, Chute DJ, Roberson ED, Pace-Savitsky C, Neumann M, Chow TW, Rosen HJ, Forstl H, Kurz A, Miller BL. Frontotemporal lobar degeneration: demographic characteristics of 353 patients. *Arch Neurol.* 2005;62:925-930.

Kawas CH. Early Alzheimers' disease. *N Engl J Med.* 2003;349:1056-63

Kertesz A. Progress in clinical neurosciences: frontotemporal dementia-Pick's disease. *Can J Neurol Sci.* 2006;33:141-148

Kipps GM, Hodges JR. Cognitive assessment for clinicians. *J Neurol Neurosurg Psychiatry.* 2005;76(suppl 1):22-30

Knibb JA, Hodges JR. Semantic dementia and primary progressive aphasia: a problem of recategorization? *Alzheimer Dis Assoc Disord.* 2005;19(Suppl 1):7-14.

Knopman DS, DeKosky ST, Cummuings JL, Chui H, Corey-Bloom J, Relkin N. Small GW, Miller B, Stevens JC. Practice parameter: Diagnosis of dementia (an evidence-based review). Report of the Quality Standards Subcommittee of the American Academy of Neurology. *Neurology.* 2001;56:1143-53

Kral VA. Senescence forgetfulness: benign and malignant. *Can Med Assoc J.* 1962;86:257-60

Langa KM, Foster L, Larson EB. Mixed dementia: Emerging concepts and therapeutic implications. *J Am Med Assoc.* 2004;292:2901-8

Laureys S, Goldman S, Phillips C, Van Bogaert P, Aerts J, Luxen A, Franck G, Maquet P. Impaired effective cortical connectivity in vegetative state. *Neuroimage.* 1999;9:377-82.

Lee HB, Lyketsos CJ. Depression in Alzheimer's disease: heterogeneity and related issues. *Biol Psychiatry.* 2003;54:353-62

Lopez OL, Becker JT, Somsak D, Dew MA, Dekorsky ST. Awareness of cognitive deficit in probabile Alzheimer's disease. *Eur Neurol.* 1993;34:277-82

Lustig C, Snyder AZ, Ghakta M, O'Brien KC, McAvoy M, Raichle ME, Morris JC, Buckner RL. Functional deactivations: change with age and dementia of the Alzheimer type. *Proc Natl Acad Sci.* 2003;100:14504-9.

Mahapatra RK, Edwards MJ, Schott JM, Bhatia KP. Corticobasal degeneration. *Lancet Neurol.* 2004;3:736-743

Mayeaux R, Sano M. Treatment of Alzheimer's disease. *N Engl J Med.* 1999;341:1670-9

McKeith IG, Galasko D, Kosaka K, Perry EK, Dickson DW, Hansen LA, Salmon DP, Lowe J, Mirra SS, Byrne EJ, Lennox G, Quinn NP, Edwardson JA, Ince PG, Bergeron C, Burns A, Miller BL, Lovestone S, Colerton D, Jansen ENH, Ballard C, de Vos RAI, Wilcock GK, Jellinger KA, Perry RH. Consensus guidelines for the clinical and pathologic diagnosis of dementia with Lewy bodies (DLB): report of the consortium on DLB international workshop. *Neurology.* 1996;47:1113-24.

McKhann GM, Albert MS, Grossman M, Miller B, Dickson D, Trojanowski JQ. Clinical and pathological diagnosis of frontotemporal dementia. *Arch Neurol* 2001;58:1803-9

McKhann G, Drachman D, Folstein M, Katzman R, Price D, Stadlan EM. Clinical diagnosis of Alzheimer's disease: report of the NINCDS-ADRDA Work Group under the auspices of Department of Health and Human Services Task Force on Alzheimer's disease. *Neurology.* 1984;34:939-44.

Migliorelli R, Teson A, Sabe L, Petracca G, Petracchi M, Leiguarda R, Starkstein SE. Anosognosia in Alzheimer's disease: a study of associated factors. *J Neuropsychiatry Clin Neurosci.* 1995;7:338-44

Miller BL, Seeley WW, Mychack P, Rosen HJ, Mena M, Boone K. Neuronatomy of the self. Evidence from patients with frontotemporal dementia. *Neurology.* 2001;57:817-21

Minoshima S, Giordani B, Berent S, Frey KA, Foster NL, Kuhl DE. Metabolic reduction in the posterior cingulate cortex in very early Alzheimer's disease. *Ann Neurol.* 1997;42:85-94.

Neary D, Snowden JS, Gustafson L, Passant U, Stuss D, Black S, Freedman M, Kertesz A, Robert PH, Albert M, Boone K, Miller BL, Cummings J, Benson DF. Frontotemporal lobar degeneration: a consensus on clinical diagnostic criteria. *Neurology.* 1998;51:1546-54.

Orgogozo JM, Gilman S, Dartigues JF, Laurent B, Puel M, Kirby LC, Jouanny P, Dubois B, Eisner L, Flitman S, Michel BF, Boada M, Frank A, Hock C. Subacute meningoencephalitis in a subset of patients with AD after Abeta42 immunization. *Neurology.* 2003;61:46-54

Ott BR, Lafleche G, Whelihan WM, Buongiorno GW, Albert MS, Fogel BS. Impaired awareness of deficits in Alzheimer's Disease. *Alzheimer Dis Assoc Dis.* 1996;10:68-76.

Padovani A, Borrioni B, Colciaghi F, Pettenati C, Cottini E, Agosti C, Lenzi GL, Caltagirone C, Trabucchi M, Cattabeni F, Di Luca M. Abnormalities in the pattern of platelet amyloid precorsor protein forms in patients with Mild Cognitive Impairment and Alzheimer's disease. *Arch Neurol.* 2002;59:71-5

Palmer AM, Stratmann GC, Procter AW, Bowen DM. Possible neutransmitter basis of behavioural changes in Alzheimers's disease. *Ann Neurol.* 1988;23:616-20

Parsons CJ, Danysz W, Quack G. Memantine is a clinically well tolerated N-methyl-D-aspartate receptor antagonist – review of preclinical data. *Neuropharmacology.* 1999;38:735-67

Parvizi J, Van Hoesen GW, Buckwalter JA, Damasio A. Neural connections of the posteromedial cortex in the macaque. *Proc Natl Acad Sci USA.* 2006;103:1563-8.

Petersen RC, Smith CE, Waring SC, Ivnik RJ, Tangalos EG, Kokmen E. Mild Cognitive Impairment: clinical characterization and outcome. *Arch Neurol.* 1999;56:303-8

Petersen RC. Mild Cognitive Impairment as a diagnostic entity. *J Intern Med.* 2004;256:183-94

Raichle ME, MacLeod AM, Snyder AZ, Powers WJ, Gusnard DA, Shulman GL. A default mode of brain function. *Proc Natl Acad Sci USA.* 2001;98:676-82.

Reiman EM, Caselli RJ, Yun LS, Chen K, Bandy D, Minoshima S, Thibodeau SN, Osborne D. Preclinical evidence of Alzheimer's disease in persons homozygous for the epsilon 4 allele for apolipoprotein E. *N Engl J Med.* 1996;334:752-8.

Reisberg B, Borenstein J, Salob SP, Ferris SH, Franssen E, Georgotas A. Behavioral symptoms in Alzheimer's disease: phenomenology and treatment. *J Clin Psychiatry.* 1987;48 (Suppl):9-15.

Richards SS, Hendrie HC. Diagnosis, management, and treatment of Alzheimer's disease. *Arch Intern Med.* 1999;159:789-98

Ritchie K, Touchon J. Mild cognitive impairment: conceptual basis and current neurological status. *Lancet.* 2000;355:255-8

Roman GC, Tatemichi TK, Erkinjuntti T, Cummings JL, Masdeu JL, Garcia JH, Amaducci L, Orgogozo JM, Brun A, Hofman A. Vascular dementia: diagnostic criteria for research studies. Report of the NINDS-AIREN International Workshop. *Neurology.* 1993;43:250-60.

Roskies A. Neuroscientific challenge to free will and responsability. *Trends Cogn Sci.* 2006;10:419-23

Rub U, Del Tredici K, Del Turco D, Braak H. The intralaminar nuclei assigned to the medial pain system and other components of this system are early and progressively affected by the Alzheimer's disease-related cytoskeletal pathology. *J Chem Neuroanat.* 2002;23:279-90.

Salmon E, Ruby P, Perani D, Kalbe E, Laureys S, Adam S, Collette F. Two aspects of impaired consciousness in Alzheimer's disease. *Prog Brain Res* 2005;150:287-98

Scahill RI, Schott JM, Stevens JM, Fox NC. Mapping the evolution of regional atrophy in Alzheimer's disease: unbiased analysis of fluid-registered serial MRI. *Proc Natl Acad Sci USA.* 2002;99:4703-7.

Schenk D, Barbour R, Dunn W, Gordon G, Grajeda H, Guido T, Hu K, Huang J, Johnson-Wood K, Khan K, Kholodenko D, Lee M, Liao Z, Lieburburg I, Motter R, Mutter L, Soriano F, Shopp G, Vasquez N, Vandevert C, Walker S, Wogulis M, Yednock T, Games D, Seubert P. Immunization with amyloid-beta attenuates Alzheimer's disease-like pathology in the PDAPP mouse. *Nature.* 1999;400:173-7

Sowell ER, Thompson PM, Holmes CJ, Batth R, Jernigan TL, Toga AW. Locakized age-related changes in brain structure between childhood and adolescence using statistical parametric mapping. *Neuroimage.* 1999;9:587-97

Squire LR. Memory and the hippocampus: a synthesis from findings with rats, monkeys and humans. *Psychol Rev.* 1992;99:195-231

Starkstein SE, Jorge R. Dementia after traumatic brain injury. *Int Psychogeriatr* 2005;17(Suppl 1):93-107

Stern RG, Duffelmeyer ME, Zemishlani Z, Davidson M. The use of benzodiazepines in the management of behavioural symptoms in dementia patients. *Psychiatr Clin North Am.* 1991;14:375-84

Strittmatter WJ, Roses AD. Apolipoproten E and Alzheimer's disease. *Proc Natl Acad Sci USA.* 1995;92:4725-7

Sturm VE, Rosen HJ, Allison S, Miller BL, Levenson RW. Self-conscious emotion deficits in frontotemporal lobe degeneration. *Brain.* 2006; 129:2508-16

Stuss DT, Benson DF. *The frontal lobes.* Raven Press, New York 1986

Talbot PR, Lloyd JJ, Snowden JS, Neary D, Testa HJ. A clinical role for 99m Tc-HMPAO SPECT in the investigation of dementia? *J Neurol Neurosurg Psychiatry.* 1998;64:306-13

Van der Flier WM, Scheltens P. Epidemiology and risk factors of dementia. *J Neurol Neurosurg Psychiatry.* 2005;76(suppl V):2-7

Van Horn JD. The new perspectives in fMRI research award: exploring patterns of default-mode brain activity. *J Cogn Neurosci.* 2004;16:1479-80.

Vasterling JJ, Seltzer B, Watrous WE. Longitudinal assessment of deficit unawareness in Alzheimer's disease. *Neuropsychiatry Neuropsychol Behav Neurol.* 1997;10:197-202

Woods RT, Moniz-Cook E, Iliffe S, Campion P, Vernooij-Dassen M, Zanetti O, Franco M. Dementia: issues in early recognition and intervention in primary care. *J Royal Soc Med.* 2003;320-4

Yaari R, Corey-Bloom J. Alzheimer's disease. *Semin Neurol.* 2007;27:32-41

Zanetti O, Vallotti B, Frisoni GB, Geroldi C, Bianchetti A, Pasqualetti P, Trabucchi. Insight in dementia: when does it occur? Evidence for a non-linear relationship between insight and cognitive status. *J Gerontol B Psychol Sci Soc Sci.* 1999;54:100-6

Zeman AZ, Grayling AC, Cowey A. Contemporary theories of consciousness. *J Neurol Neurosurg Psychiatry.* 1997;62:549-52

Chapter 7

THE FRAGMENTED SELF: DISSOCIATIVE DISORDERS

Who over certain things does not lose his mind, he has no mind to lose at all

Emilia Galotti, by Gotthold Ephraim Lessing (1772)

7.1. PSYCHIATRY AND CONSCIOUSNESS

The alterations of consciousness in psychiatric disease have been matter of huge debate in the XX century, especially by French and German authors (see Ey 1963, for extensive review). Given the objective difficulties in formulating a consensus-based operational definition of the concept of "consciousness", in the most recent American and European classifications (DSM-IV and ICD-10, respectively) disorders of consciousness are marginally described or even not described at all as specific syndromic entities.

The first methodological issue to face in this field is probably the one concerning descriptive terminology, as psychiatric literature employs a wide range of denominative, interpretative, qualitative and quantitative terms that may often generate perplexity and increase rather than decrease confusion (Table 7.1).

In the present chapter we will focus on dissociative disorders, i.e. the category of psychiatric disturbances of current diagnostic nosology which includes a wide variety of syndromes whose common core is an alteration of consciousness affecting memory and identity as well.

Dissociation is a fascinating and obscure neuropsychiatric phenomenon, described as one of the least explored frontiers in psychobiology (Simeon 2004). It is defined by DSM-IV-TR (1994) as a disruption of the usually integrated functions of consciousness, memory, identity or perception of the environment, leading to a fragmentation of the coherence, unity and continuity of the sense of self. Dissociative experiences may occur in a continuum of situations, from healthy individuals, often under conditions of stress, fatigue or drug abuse, to a severely debilitating disorder where symptoms can persist chronically and unremittingly for decades. They have been described in a number of neurological conditions (e.g. epilepsy and migraine), but most commonly present within the context of psychiatric disorders, especially anxiety disorders (panic disorder) and depression (Hunter et al. 2004). The group of dissociative disorders include an extraordinary set of conditions, such as dissociative amnesia, dissociative fugue, dissociative identity disorder (formerly multiple personality disorder), and depersonalization disorder, in which what is normally a unified conscious experience undergoes all kinds of schisms and fractures. Other psychiatric disorders, such as schizophrenia, may also share some traits with dissociative disorders *qua* disorders of neural integration. However, what follows concerns dissociative conditions *sensu strictu,* as defined by current psychiatric nosography.

Table 7.1. Terms most commonly used in psychiatry to describe the psychopathology of consciousness

Altered states of consciousness	*Aspecific term used to indicate "all the variations of the normal conditions of consciousness"*
States of obnubilation	*Quantitative alterations of consciousness (level of general awareness)*
Crepuscular states	*"Narrowing of consciousness", with hyporeactivity to external stimuli and hallucinatory and delusional production*
Dreamy states	*Similar to crepuscular states*
Hypnoid states	*Similar to states of obnubilation, a term derived from the normal transition phase from wakening to sleep*
Onyric, amential or confusional states	*Similar to "delirium"*
Dissociation	*Severe alteration of the normally integrated functions of consciousness, memory, identity or perception of the environment*

In the ICD-10 classification (1992), dissociative ("conversion") disorders cover a range of signs and symptoms previously ascribed to the old concept of "hysteria", whereas DSM-IV allocates them as conversion disorders in the somatoform disorders category. This difference, along with a series of other inconsistencies, well illustrate the confusion that surrounds the definition of dissociation in contemporary psychiatric nosography (Holmes et al. 2005; Kihlstrom 2001). Furthermore, post-traumatic stress disorder (PTSD) is not categorized by either DSM-IV-TR or ICD-10, although symptoms of dissociation are reported by several patients with PTSD (Ehlers and Clark 2000). A recent 1-year prospective study following the 9/11 World Trade Center disaster revealed a strong association of baseline dissociation with dissociative experiences at follow-up (Simeon et al. 2004).

Two main conceptual approaches have been proposed for a thorough understanding of the causes of dissociative disorders. The first one is exemplified by PTSD, as stated above, whereas the second one explains the proneness to experience dissociative symptoms within the context of normal personality traits, including (among others) hypnotizability, mental "absorption" and tendency to fantasize (Isaac and Chand 2006).

7.2. DISSOCIATIVE AMNESIA

Dissociative (or psychogenic) amnesia is typically retrograde, and entails a loss of personal memory that cannot be accounted for by ordinary forgetting, traumatic brain injury or other neurological diseases (Kopelman 1987). It can be *localized*, i.e. circumscribed to a given period of time; *selective*, i.e. only for certain events; more rarely *generalized* (for the entire past life of the subject) or *continuative* (from a given moment to present time).

Dissociative amnesia is often encountered in victims of violent crime or people involved in catastrophic events, thus representing a symptom of PTSD. However, it is also frequently claimed by perpetrators of violent crimes. A well-known example is the case of the Palestinian terrorist Sirhan Sirhan, who on June 4, 1968 shot and killed Senator Robert F. Kennedy in Los Angeles, California. He was unable to remember this event following his arrest. However, when hypnotized, Sirhan was eventually able to recall and even reenact the episode, but these memories were not accessible to him after hypnosis was terminated (Diamond, 1980). Although psychogenic amnesia has been the frequent subject of popular treatises, there has been very little scientifically-ground research on the nature of the memory loss, its eliciting conditions, and the circumstances that lead to recovery of the lost memories.

7.3. DISSOCIATIVE FUGUE

Psychogenic fugue (otherwise called *functional retrograde amnesia*) combines the loss of personal memory (as observed in psychogenic amnesia) with the loss of identity, and sometimes physical relocation (Kihlstrom 2001). Moreover, in psychogenic fugue the precipitating event is usually a physical or mental trauma - or a severe depressive episode. The process of recovery from fugue is still unclear. Some patients experience a sudden awakening to their original identity, while others experience a sudden awareness that they do not know who they are. Nevertheless, upon recovery the patient is typically left with an island of amnesia covering the period of the fugue state. It has been hypothesized that during fugue episodes a selective disruption in memory occurs, technically a dissociation (Schachter and Tulving 1982): episodic memory (which relates to episodes of personal experience) is impaired, whilst semantic memory (i.e. general knowledge about facts and notions) is spared.

It should be mentioned that the distinction between psychogenic fugue and psychogenic amnesia is often difficult to make. While one might say that fugues are simply very generalized amnesias, the loss of identity that is pathognomic of fugue may represent a qualitative difference.

7.4. DEPERSONALIZATION DISORDER

Depersonalization is a particular type of dissociation involving a disrupted integration of self-perception/sense of self, such that individuals experiencing depersonalization subjectively feel estranged, detached or disconnected from their own being. Experiences of depersonalization were originally described as co-occurring with the ones of derealization (Mayer-Gross 1935). It was believed that depersonalization was the expression of a pre-formed brain response of life-threatening events or a "pre-forced" brain response similar to delirium, catatonia, seizures etc. More recently, depersonalization and derealization have been conceptualized as separate entities, with the suggestion that derealization is the more general case, and depersonalization is a limited form, in which only the experience of self is altered (Nemiah 1989). The DSM-IV (American Psychiatric Association 1994) more properly defines depersonalization as "a feeling of detachment or estrangement from one's self" and includes among the defining criteria "a sensation of being an outside observer of one's body and feeling like an automaton or as if (one) is living in a dream". Derealization, on the other hand, refers to "an alteration in the perception of one's surroundings so that a sense of reality of the external world is lost". Both depersonalization and derealization are frequently observed as symptoms of other psychiatric syndromes, such as anxiety, depression and obsession (Trueman 1984; Mula et al. 2006a), and they are salient components in the near-death experiences reported by people rescued from drownings, falls or other kinds of severe accidents (Noyes and Kletti 1977). Moreover, depersonalization is usually accompanied by a state of hyperalertness and enhanced sensory processing. However, depersonalization and derealization also constitute autonomous syndromes. In this case, the main feature of this syndrome is a subjective awareness of feeling of change in oneself (depersonalization) or the world (derealization). Although these feelings may be pleasant when self-induced by means of yoga meditation, psychedelic drugs, in clinical cases they are characteristically unpleasant. The subject retains insight into what is happening throughout the episode. Distorsions of sensation and perception, changes in the experience of personal time, enhanced memory for the personal past experiences and changes in body image are commonly experienced. Cognitive impairments are frequent, specifically a decline in the ability to focus on complex tasks, increased forgetfulness in daily life activities and difficulty in vividly evoking past memories. Accordingly, specific attention and memory deficts have been demonstrated with neuropsychiatric testing (Guralnik et al. 2000).

Depersonalization, derealization, déjà-vu and-jamais vu experiences occur also in patients with epilepsy – see also chapter 5 (Alvarez-Silva et al. 2006). Although the interest in their phenomenology and epidemiology has flourished over the last decades with the accumulation of a large literature, they have been only occasionally investigated in patients with epilepsy, because researchers focused their attention mainly on patients with pseudoseizures (i.e. non epileptic attacks). An interesting study by Devinsky et al. (1989), showed that scores at the specific Dissociative Experience Scale (DES) (Bernstein et al. 1986) in seizure patients were moderately elevated compared with those of healthy individuals, but similar to those reported for psychiatric patients with anxiety or phobic disorders. More recently, a study by the authors of this volume (Mula et al. 2006b) demonstrated no difference in DES scores among patients with or without epileptic auras or in different aura subtype (especially psychic), suggesting that dissociative experiences experienced by patients with epilepsy are not likely to be related to the aura itself. However, DES scores correlated with the anxiety subscale (ANX) of the Minnesota Multiphasic Personality Inventory MMPI-2 (Hathaway and McKinley 1989) and the state subscale of the State-Trait Anxiety Inventory (STAI-Y2, Spielberger 1983) only in patients with aura. Taken together, these results seem to suggest that dissociative experiences in epilepsy rarely represent true epileptic phenomena but are usually associated with anxiety symptomatology. These findings have theoretical relevance in the light of the current concept of dissociation in epilepsy (Brown and Trimble 2000). The notion that several epileptic phenomena can be regarded as dissociative experiences is often based on the occurrence of amnesia (Good 1993), but several manifestations associated with partial seizures, such as cognitive auras, déja vu, déja vécu, jamais vu and others should be distinguished from true episodes of dissociation, based on the pathogenesis. Auras probably originate from the activation of highly vivid representational structures within the temporal lobes, either directly by seizure activity in representational networks, or indirectly through seizure-related stimulation of limbic structures, such as the amygdala and the anterior cingulate (Brown 2002).

7.5. DISSOCIATIVE IDENTITY DISORDER

In dissociative identity disorder (DID), formerly defined as *multiple personality disorder*, an individual appears to manifest two or more distinct identities. Each personality alternates in control over conscious experience, thought and action, and is separated from the other(s) by some degree of amnesia (Wilkes 1988).

More than one thousand cases have been described so far. Most cases are anecdoctal ones, and single-case studies using both experimental and psychometric methods have been somewhat rarer. A good half of the patients would have more than ten personalities; many subjects would be erroneously diagnosed as affected by schizophrenia or borderline personality disorder. In recent literature, particular relevance in their causative mechanisms is given to child trauma (especially sexual abuse), and, to a lesser extent, military combat and satanic rituals. However, there is much controversy about the real prevalence of DID, with huge discrepancies between American and European psychiatrists (Putnam 1991). These last ones believe that DID might be an artifactual phenomen, especially induced by hypnosis (Gelder and Gath 1996). The syndrome is certainly more frequent in women (75-90% of the cases) (Andreasen and Black 1991), and might represent up to 3-5% of all psychiatric diagnoses (Kaplan and Sadock 1995).

The influence of interpersonal, cultural, and historical factors on DID can hardly be denied, but it is also something of a puzzle. The fact that the diagnosis experienced a golden age, waned after 1920, and showed a resurgence of in the 1970s makes one wonder about the social conditions in which dissociative behaviors are expressed, and corresponding diagnoses made. Furthermore, especially in view of the virtual avalanche of cases reported in both the professional and popular over the past decades, it is quite surprising that so few cases have been subject to experimental analysis under controlled conditions.

More recently, neurophysiological, psychophysiological and psychometric techniques have been employed to differentiate DID from other dissociative disorders and disturbances in patients with epilepsy and pseudoseizures (Bowman and Coons 2000; Mula et al. 2006b), suggesting that misdiagnosis of people with seizures and dissociative symptoms can be avoided by using video-EEG monitoring and systematic assessment of dissociative symptoms with specific scales (e.g. the DES), and the Structured Clinical Interview for DSM-IV Dissociative Disorders, SCID-D (Steinberg 1994).

7.6. HYSTERIA

Hysteria, a nosological term no longer employed in modern official diagnostic classifications, which probably requires description and eventually reconsideration in the context of consciousness studies (Creed 2006). "Hysteria" is a word derived from the Greek word for "uterus" and was originally coined by Hippocrates, who thought that the condition occurred only in women and it was caused by movements of the uterus in the body. This is not the proper place to go deeply into the history and evolution of the concept of hysteria across the centuries, which has continuously fascinated both clinicians and theorists interested in altered states of self-consciousness (Mai 1995). Anyway, it should be mentioned that our understanding of hysteria as a psychiatric condition mostly relies on the classic study by Pierre Briquet (1859) and even more on those by Jean-Martin Charcot (1892) and by his scholars (especially Babinski, Janet, and Richer) performed at the Salpêtrière Hospital in Paris during the second half of the XIX century.

It must also be remembered that Freud's earliest psychoanalytic works on hysteria were strongly influenced by Charcot's theories (Knight 1984).

Currently, hysteria is referred to as a "conversion disorder" (DSM-IV 1994), that is not explained by an organic neurological lesion or medical disease, arising in relation to some psychological stress or conflict, but not consciously produced or intentionally feigned. This disorder belongs to the category of *somatoform disorders,* along with somatization disorder, hypochondria, somatoform (psychogenic) pain disorder, body dysmorphic disorder (formerly known as dysmorphophobia) and the like.

Among the symptoms of hysteria, dissociative (or psychogenic) amnesia (see paragraph 7.2) is the one most closely related to alterations of consciousness, but it is much rarer than previously thought, whereas conversion represents the most common feature. The nature and character of the most representative symptoms embrace the whole field of clinical neurology: weakness, paralyses, sensory disturbances, pseudoseizures and involuntary movements (e.g. tremor) (Pryse-Phyllips and Murray 1992). After more than a century of intense clinical and theoretical debate, all modern theories of conversion acknowledge the fact that a primary psychological disturbance is probably responsible for triggering subjective physical symptoms, and perhaps also for triggering some associated changes in the neurophysiological state of the central nervous system (for extensive review, see Vuilleumier 2005). However, the exact nature of the emotional disorders responsible for hysterical symptoms, and their functional consequences on neural systems in the brain, still remain largely unknown. Several studies have used neurophysiological and functional brain imaging techniques (EEG, scalp evoked potentials, motor evoked potentials, fMRI, PET, or SPECT) in order to diagnose hysteria (i.e., to exclude neurological deficits) (Cantello et al. 2001; Drake 1990; Lorenz et al. 1998), or to identify specific neural correlates associated with hysterical conversion symptoms (Broome 2004). Vuilleumier et al. (2001) first investigated the neural correlates of conversion disorder by showing hypoactivity of the basal ganglia and the thalamus, in a rigorous imaging study further supported by volumetric investigations (Atmaca et al. 2006). These selective activation abnormalities are intriguing, since these regions are interconnected into functional loops forming a cortico-striato-thalamo-cortical circuit which is critical for voluntary motor action. Moreover, the striatum (especially the caudate nucleus) represents an essential neural site within such loops where motivational signals can modulate motor preparation activity (Alexander et al. 1986; Haber 2003). Similar studies have revealed selective decreases in the activity of frontal and subcortical circuits involved in motor control during hysterical paralysis, decreases in somatosensory cortex during hysterical anesthesia, or decreases in visual cortex during hysterical blindness (Black et al. 2004; Marshall et al. 1997; Tiihonen et al. 1995; Vuilleumier 2005). On the other hand, other studies have shown increased activation in limbic regions, such as cingulate or orbitofrontal cortex during conversion symptoms affecting different sensory or motor modalities (Konishi et al. 1999; Paus 2001).

Taken together, these data generally do not support previous proposals that hysteria might involve an exclusion of sensorimotor representation from awareness to attentional processes, but rather seem to suggest a modulation of such representations by primary affective or stress-related factors, perhaps involving primitive reflexive mechanisms of protection and alertness that are partly independent of conscious control, and seem to be mediated by dynamic modulatory interactions between limbic and sensorimotor networks (Krem 2004; Trimble 1996; Vuilleumier 2005).

7.7. THE NEUROBIOLOGY OF DEPERSONALIZATION

A number of neurochemical studies have been conducted on subjects with depersonalization, as this disorder can be caused by different psychoactive agents. The four classes of substances implicated in the induction of depersonalisation states in healthy controls are glutamate NMDA receptor antagonists, cannabinoids, hallucinogens, and opiod receptor agonists.

The NMDA antagonist ketamine, also known as the "dissociative anesthetic", can induce profound dissociative states in healthy individuals, quite similarly to the negative symptoms of schizophrenia (Curran and Morgan 2000). It is possible that diminished NMDA-related neurotransmission is related to the dissociative states, as NMDA receptors are widely distributed in the cortex, as well as in the hippocampus and the amygdala, and are thought to mediate associative functioning and long-term potentiation of memory (Holt 1997).

Cannabinoids, such as marijuana, have also been shown to induce depersonalization in healthy individuals (Simeon et al. 2003). A positron emission tomography (PET) study using intravenous tetrahydrocannabinol found that the severity of depersonalization symptomatology correlated with increased cerebral blood flow in the right frontal cortex and the anterior cingulate, and decreased subcortical blood flow in the amygdala, hippocampus, basal ganglia, and thalamus (Mathew et al. 1999). In addition to their action on cannabinoid receptors, cannabinoids have been shown to block NMDA receptors at sites distinct from other noncompetitive NMDA antagonists (Feigenbaum et al. 1989), thus suggesting that their dissociative effect might be mediated via the NMDA receptor.

Depersonalization states in healthy individuals can be transiently induced by the use of hallucinogens, such as lysergide (LSD), psylocybine and dimethyltryptamine (Simeon et al. 2003b). These substances act as agonists on serotonin 5-HT 2A and 5-HT2C receptors, thus suggesting a possible mediating role of serotonin in depersonalization. A study with the 5-HT2C receptor agonist meta-chlorophenylpiperazine (m-CPP) demonstrated the induction of depersonalization in patients with different psychiatric diagnoses (social phobia, borderline personality disorder and obsessive compulsive disorder) (Simeon et al. 1995), while dissociative symptoms were induced in a subgroup of patients with posttraumatic stress disorder (Southwick et al. 1997). A PET imaging study showed that the hallucinogenic 5HT 1A/2A receptor agonist psylocibine resulted in increased dopamine in the striatum that correlated with depersonalization (Vollenweider et al. 1999).

In healthy individuals, the k-opiod agonist enadoline has been demonstrated to induce a depersonalization-like syndrome compared with placebo (Walsh et al., 2001). Conversely, opioid antagonists such as high dose naltrexone and intravenous naloxone have been shown to reduce dissociation in psychiatric patients (Bohus et al. 1996; Nuller et al. 2001).

There is limited but compelling evidence for autonomic hyporeactivity in depersonalization disorder: in a study comparing skin conductance response to unpleasant stimuli in healthy individuals and patients with anxiety disorders (Sierra et al. 2002b), patients with depersonalization disorder demonstrated a selective inhibition of emotional processing. Noradrenaline has been proposed as the neurotransmitter playing the central role in this inhibition (Simeon et al. 2003a). In addition, the hypothalamic-pituitary-adrenal axis (HPA) seems to contribute in mediating the stress response, and there is extensive evidence for its sensitization in PTSD (Yehuda 1997). HPA axis dysregulation may occur in depersonalization disorders, but currently available data are conflicting (Simeon et al. 2001; Stanton et al. 2001).

7.8. THE NEURAL CORRELATES OF DISSOCIATION

The pioneering studies by Penfield and Rasmussen (1950) in patients undergoing cortical stimulation of the superior and middle temporal gyri, and experiencing derealization-like states, led the authors to think that these perceptual phenomena could be produced "only in the temporal region, perhaps extending somehow to the occipital cortex". More recently, a "corticolimbic disconnection hypothesis" has been proposed (Sierra and Berrios 1998), with prefrontal activation and limbic inhibition, resulting in hypoemotionality (via amygdalar inhibition) as well as attentional difficulties (via cingulate inhibition). There seem to be two distinct components of the depersonalization experience subsumed by distinct brain circuitries: visual derealization is associated with occipito-temporal dysfunction, and body alienation is associated with parietal function (Sierra et al. 2002a).

The integration of different cortical areas might be necessary for cohesive conscious experience, and this intracortical connectivity might be NMDA-receptor mediated, and hence blocked by ketamine (see paragraph 7.7) (Krystal et al. 1998). Dissociation might therefore involve the disruption of corticocortical, thalamocortical, amygdalocortical and hippocampocortical networks.

As the subjective sense of "unfamiliarity" is crucial to the depersonalization experience, an incoming perception not processed as familiar will be experienced as unreal, strange and detached. It is likely, therefore, that the primary alterations underlying depersonalization (and derealization) may lie in brain areas responsible for matching incoming sensory information to pre-existing memory networks related to these perceptions, thus involving both limbic structures and sensory association cortical areas.

In a study using fMRI with traumatic script-driven imagery, women with PTSD secondary to childhood sexual abuse experienced dissociative states (occurring in 30% of subjects) while neuroimaging showed an increase activation in the medial prefrontal cortex, inferior frontal gyrus, anterior cingulate, superior and middle temporal gyri, parietal and occipital lobe (Lanius et al. 2002). In another fMRI study the responses to neutral and aversive visual stimuli were compared across three groups: 1) patients with depersonalization disorder; 2) patients with obsessive-compulsive disorder and 3) healthy controls. Patients with depersonalization disorder rated the aversive pictures as less emotive than those with obsessive-compulsive disorder, and their insula (part of the limbic system that is involved in disgust sensation) was not activated, unlike individuals in the other two groups (Phillips et al. 2001). Furthermore, patients with depersonalization disorder showed increased activation in the right ventral prefrontal cortex, thus suggesting that the neural mechanism for emotional detachment might be mediated by prefrontal activation and limbic inhibition.

In a PET and MRI study (Simeon et al. 2000), patients with depersonalization disorder exhibited stronger left-sided laterality than healthy controls, with significantly different overall patterns of activity in the posterior cortex (temporal, parietal and occipital lobes). More precisely, lower activity in the right temporal region (Brodmann areas 21 and 22), higher activity in the parietal region bilaterally (areas 7 and 39) and higher activity in left occipital region (area 19), all of these areas being components of the sensory cortex. Brodmann area 22 is an auditory association area; area 19 is a visual association area; area 7 is a somatosensory association and area 39 (the angular gyrus) is a multimodal associative area strategically located in the inferior parietal lobule, a region that receives sensory input from the parietal, temporal and occipital cortices, and therefore is central to a well-integrated body schema. Taken together, these data indicate that depersonalization disorder may be related to disrupted functioning along hierarchical sensory association areas responsible for the processing of incoming perceptions against pre-existing brain templates.

Moreover, it is likely that the components and dimensions of depersonalization are differentially controlled by the right and left hemisphere. Data on the interactions between laterality and depersonalization are contradictory: Devinsky et al. (1989) reported higher scores for the DES depersonalization subscale in subjects with partial epilepsy affecting the dominant hemisphere, whereas Smirnov (1977) suggested that patients with space-occupying lesions in the right temporal lobe are more related to report depersonalisation experiences.

Overall, it is clear that knowledge about the neurobiology of emotions represents an important component for the understanding of depersonalization. The assessment of emotional significance seems to be an unconscious process (Halgren and Marinkovic 1994), and the fact that feelings of immediacy and vividness seem to accompany perceptions that are fragmentary and cognitively underprocessed (as those generated by amygdala stimulation), also supports the view that emotional feelings play a crucial role in the way reality is experienced. According to this view, disruption of the process that affectively colors cognition and perception imposes a qualitative change on the subjective experience, which is then reported as a lack of vividness or a feeling of unreality (Sierra and Berrios 2002).

7.9. FUNCTIONAL NEUROIMAGING OF CONVERSION

The aforementioned studies in conversion disorders have indicated a possible interruption of motor command with volition being intact. As it is known, motor command is mediated by cingulate activation in conjunction with orbitofrontal cortex, with the anterior cingulate being an interface between limbic and neocortical functions. Cingulate activation reflects the degree of intentional effort needed to carry out a task (Winterer et al. 2002). Other studies have rather suggested the possibility of a deficit of volition and dysfunction of the left dorsolateral prefrontal cortex. In a fMRI study (Mailis-Gagnon et al. 2003) in conversion disorder patients, different areas of activation were detected in response to sensory stimulation, i.e. anterior insula, thalamus, caudal anterior cingulate cortex and ventrolateral prefrontal cortex. The authors suggested the possibility of functional deafferentation due to active inhibition of somatosensory processing by limbic areas.

Studies conducted in hypnotically paralysed subjects have shown increased activation in right anterior cingulate, orbitofrontal cortex and right posterior medial orbitofrontal cortex (Halligan et al. 2000; Ward et al. 2003). These results lead the authors to speculate that the primary deficit lies in motor initiation, with volition being intact. In their opinion, orbitofrontal cortex modulates the interaction of behavioural and emotional inhibition.

All these studies support the hypothesis that dissociative disorders, and specifically the ones characterized by conversion symptoms, result from the dynamic reorganization of neural circuits that link volition, movement and perception. Disruption in this network may occur in the stage of preconscious motor planning and modality-specific attention, as suggested by the right frontoparietal network subserving self-regulation and the affective correlates of selfhood (Blake et al. 2004)

7.10. CONSCIOUSNESS IN PSYCHOANALYSIS

It is universally known that the major "Freudian" revolution consisted in the so called "discovery of the unconscious" (Ellenberger 1979), as Sigmund Freud divided the psychological phenomena in *conscious, preconscious* and *unconscious* ones. Freud considered consciousness as the mere surface of psychic life, developing in his own original way the assumptions of the philosopher Leibniz (Mates 1986) and the psychiatrist Janet (1894) on the existence of non conscious elementary perceptions .

It is far beyond the aims of this chapter to go through the details of Freud's theories, as well as the popular theories of his pupils and followers, including Carl Gustav Jung, Alfred Adler, Melaine Klein, from the very beginning of psychoanalysis to our times. A number of treatises provide an extensive review of this subject, also including the relationship between psychoanalysis and philosophy of mind (e.g. Cavell 1993; Fonagy and Target 2003; Spector Person et al. 2003; Wollheim 1991). Quite recently, a new science called "neuropsychoanalysis" offered a re-interpretation of Freud's theories in the light of the recent discoveries in neuroscience (for an overview on the principles of neuropsychoanalysis, the reader is referred to Solms 2006). Anyway, it is mandatory to point out how, in the (allegorical) psychoanalytic view of the "theatre of the mind", consciousness plays a rather secondary role, since the *ego* (i.e. the self) appears to be squeezed in between the instinctual pressures of the unconscious (the *"es"*) and the oppressing forces of the *super-ego* (i.e. the internal moral law).

7.11. REFERENCES

Alexander GE, DeLong MR, Strick PL. Parallel organization of functionally segregated circuits linking basal ganglia and cortex. *Ann Rev Neurosci.* 1986;9:357-81

Alvarez-Silva S, Alvarez Silva I, Alvarez-Rodriguez J, Peres-Echeverria MJ, Campayo-Martinez A, Rodriguez-Fernandez FL. Epileptic consciousness: concept and meaning of aura. *Epil Behav.* 2006;8:527-33

Andreasen NC, Black DW. *Introductory textbook of Psychiatry.* American Psychiatric Press, Washington D.C., London 1991

Atmaca M, Aydin A, Tezcan E, Kursad Poyraz A, Kara B. Volumetric investigation of brain regions in patients with conversion disorder. *Prog Neuro-Psychopharmacol Biol Psychiatry.* 2006;30:708-13

Black DN, Seritan AL, Taber KH, Hurley RA. Conversion hysteria: lessons from functional imaging. *J Neuropsychiatry Clin Neurosci.* 2004;16:245-51

Bohus MJ, Landwehrmeyer GB, Stiglmayr CE, Limberger MF, Bohme R, Schmahl CG. Naltrexone in the treatment of dissociative symptoms in patients with borderline personality disorder: an open-label trial. *J Clin Psychiatry.* 1999;5:598-603

Bowman ES, Coons PM. The differential diagnosis of epilepsy, pseudoseizures, dissociative identity disorder, and dissociative disorder not otherwise specified. *Bull Menninger Clinic.* 2000;64:165-80

Briquet P. *Traitè clinique et thèrapèutique de l'hystèrie.* Bailliere, Paris 1859

Broome MR. A neuroscience of hysteria? *Curr Opin Psychiatry.* 2004;17:465-9

Brown RJ. Epilepsy, dissociation and nonepileptic seizures. In Trimble MR, Schmitz B. *The Neuropsychiatry of epilepsy.* Cambridge University Press, Cambridge 2002:189-209

Brown RJ, Trimble MR. Dissociative psychopathology, non-epileptic seizures and neurology. *J Neurol Neurosurg Psychiatry.* 2000;69:285-9

Cantello R, Boccagni C, Comi C, Civardi C, Monaco F. Diagnosis of psychogenic paralysis: the role of motor evoked potentials. *J Neurol.* 2001;248:889-97

Cavell M. *The psychoanalytic mind: from Freud to philosophy.* Harvard University Press, Cambridge, Mass. USA 1993

Charcot JM. *Leçons du mardi à la Salpetrière (1887-1888).* Bureau de Progrès Médical, Paris 1892

Creed F. Should general psychiatry ignore somatization and hypochondriasis? *World Psychiatry* 2006;5:146-150

Curran HV, Morgan G. Cognitive, dissociative and psychotogenic effects of ketamine in recreational users on the night and 3 days later. *Addiction.* 2000;95:575-90

Devinsky O, Putnam F, Grafman J, Bromfield E, Theodore WH. Dissociative states and epilepsy. *Neurology.* 1989;39:835-40

Diamond BL. Inherent problems in the use of pretrial hypnosis on a prospective witness. *California Law Rev.* 2000;68:313-49

Drake ME. Clinical utility of event related-potentials in neurology and psychiatry. *Semin Neurol.* 1990;10:196-203

Ehlers A, Clark DM. A cognitive model of posttraumatic stress disorder. *Behav Res Ther.* 2000;38:319-45

Ellenberger HF. *The discovery of the unconscious. The history and evolution of dynamic psychiatry.* Basic Books, New York 1970

Ey H. *La conscience.* P.U.F., Paris 1963

Feigenbaum JJ, Bergmann F, Richmond SA, Mechoulam R, Nadler V, Kloog Y, Sokolovsky M. Non psychotropic cannabinoid acts as a functional N-methyl-D-aspartate receptor blocker. *Proc Natl Acad Sci USA.* 1989;86:9584-7

Fonagy P, Target M. *Psychoanalytic theories: perspectives from developmental psychopathology.* Whurr Publications, London 2003

Good MI: The concept of an organic dissociative syndrome: what is the evidence? *Harv Rev Psychiatry.* 1993;1:145-57

Guralnik O, Schmeidler J, Simeon D. Feeling unreal: cognitive processes in depersonalization. *Am J Psychiatry.* 2000;157:103-9

Haber SN. The primate basal ganglia: parallel and integrative networks. *J Chem Neuroanat.* 2003;26:317-30

Halgren E, Marinkovic K. Neurophysiological networks integrating human emotions. In Gazzaniga M. *The cognitive neurosciences*, MIT Press, Cambridge, Mass. 1994:1137-51

Halligan PW, Athwal BS, Oakley DA, Frackowiak RSJ. Imaging hypnotic paralysis: implications for conversion hysteria. *Lancet.* 2000;355:986-7

Holmes EA, Brown RJ, Mansell W, Pasco Fearon R, Hunter ECM, Frasquilho F, Oakley DA. Are there two qualitatively distinct forms of dissociation? A review and some clinical implications. *Clin Psychol Rev.* 2005;25:1-23

Holt WF. Glutamate in health and disease: the role of inhibitors. In Bär PR, Flint Beal M. *Neuroprotection in CNS diseases.* Marcel Dekker, New York 1997:87-119

Hathaway S, McKinley J. *Minnesota Multiphasic Personality Inventory-2 Manual for administration and scoring.* University of Minnesota Press, Minneapolis 1989

Janet P. *L'automatisme psychologique.* Felix, Alcan 1894

Kihlstrom JF. Dissociative disorders. In Sutker PB. and Adams HE. *Comprehensive handbook of psychopathology.* Kluwer Academic/Plenum, New York 2001:259-76

Knight IF. "Freud's "Project": a theory for studies on hysteria. *J History Behav Sci.* 1984;20:340-58

Krem NM. Motor conversion disorders reviewed from a neuropsychiatric perspective. *J Clin Psychiatry.* 2004;65:783-90

Krystal J, Brenner D, Southwick SM, Charney DS. The emerging neurobiology of dissociation: implications for the treatment of posttraumatic stress disorder. In: Brenner JD, Marmar CR. *Trauma, memory and dissociation.* American Psychiatric Press, Washington D.C. 1998

Isaac M, Chand PK. Dissociative and conversion disorders: defining boundaries. *Curr Opin Psychiatry.* 2006;19:61-6

Kaplan HI, Sadock BJ. *Comprehensive Textbook of Psychiatry, 8th Ed.* Williams & Wilkins, Baltimore 2004

Konishi S, Nakajima K, Uchida I, Kikyo H, Kameyama M, Miyashita Y. Common inhibitory mechanism in human inferior prefrontal cortex revealed by event-related functional MRI. *Brain.* 1999;122:981-91

Kopelman MD. Amnesia: organic and psychogenic. *Br J Psychiatry.* 1987;150:428-42

Lanius RA, Williamson PC, Boksman K, Densmore M, Gupta M, Neufeld RW, Gati JS, Menon RS. Brain activation during script-driven imagery induced dissociative responses in PTSD: a functional magnetic resonance investigation. *Biol Psychiatry.* 2002;52:305-11

Lorenz J, Kunze K, Bromm B. Differentation of conversive sensory loss and malingering by P300 in a modified oddball task. *Neuroreport.* 1998;9:187-91

Mai FM. "Hysteria" in clinical neurology. *Can J Neurol Sci.* 1995;22:101-10

Mailis-Gagnon A, Giannoylis I, Downar J, Kwan CL, Mikulis DJ, Crawley AP, Nocholson K, Davis KD. Altered central somatosensory processing in chronic pain patients with "hysterical anesthesia". *Neurology.* 2003;60:1501-7

Marshall JC, Halligan PW, Fink GR, Wade TT, Frackowiak RSJ. The functional anatomy of a hysterical paralysis. *Cognition.* 1997;64:B1-B8

Mates B. *The philosophy of Leibniz.* Oxford University Press, Oxford 1986

Mathew RJ, Wilson WH, Chiu NY, Turkington TG, Degrado TR, Coleman RE. Regional cerebral blood flow and depersonalization after tetrahydrocannabinol administration. *Acta Psychiatr Scand.* 1999;100:67-75

Mayer-Gross W. On depersonalization. *Br J Med Psychol.* 1935;15:103-12

Mula M, Pini S, Cassano GB. The neurobiology and clinical significance of depersonalization in mood and anxiety disorders: a critical reappraisal. *J Neuropsychiatry Clin Neurosci.* 2006a;99:91-9.

Mula M, Cavanna A, Collimedaglia L, Barbagli D, Magli E, Monaco F. The role of aura and dissociative experiences in epilepsy. *J Neuropsychiatry Clin Neurosci.* 2006b;18:536-42

Nemiah JC. Dissociative disorders (hysterical neuroses, dissociative type). In Kaplan HI, Sadock BJ. *Comprehensive textbook of psychiatry,* 6th Ed., Williams & Wilkins, Baltimore 1995:1028-44

Noyes R, Kletti R. Depersonalization in response to life-threatening danger. *Comprehensive Psychiatry.* 1977;18:375-84

Nuller YL, Morozova MG, Kushnir ON, Hamper N. Effect of naloxone therapy on depersonalization: a pilot study. *J Psychopharmacol.* 2001;15:93-5

Paus T. Primate anterior cingulate cortex: where motor control, drive and cognition interface. *Nat Rev Neurosci.* 2001;2:417-24

Penfield W, Rasmussen T. *The cerebral cortex of man: a clinical study of localization of function.* MacMillan Co, New York 1990

Phillips ML, Medford N, Senior C, Bullmore ET, Suckling J, Brammer MJ, Andrew C, Sierra M, Williams SC, David AS. Depersonalization disorder: thinking without feeling. *Psychiatry Res.* 2001;108:145-60

Pryse-Phillips W, Murray TJ. *Examination for functional disorders.* In Essential Neurology, 4th Edition, Appleton & Lange, Norwalk, Conn 1992:71-8

Putnam F. Recent research on Multiple Personality Disorder. *Psychiatr Clin North Amer.* 1991;14:489-502

Schachter DL, Tulving E. Memory, amnesia and the episodic /semantic distinction. In Isaacson RL, Spear NE. (eds) *The expression of knowledge.* Plenum Press, New York 1982:33-65

Sierra M, Berrios GE. Depersonalization: neurobiological perspectives. *Biol Psychiatry.* 1998;44:898-908

Simeon D, Guralnik O, Knutelska M, Hollander E, Schmeidler J. Hypothalamic-pituitary-adrenal axis dysregulation in depersonalization disorder. *Neuropsychopharmcol.* 2001;25:793-5

Sierra M, Lopera F, Lambert MV, Phillips ML, David AS. Separating depersonalization and derealization: the relevance of the "lesion" method. *J Neurol Neurosurg Psychiatry.* 2002a;72:530-32

Sierra M, Senior C, Dalton J, McDonough M, Bond A, Phillips ML, O'Dwyer AM, David AS. Autonomic response in depersonalization disorder. *Arch Gen Psychiatry.* 2002b;9:833-8

Simeon D. Depersonalization disorder. A contemporary overview. *CNS Drugs.* 2004;18:343-54

Simeon D, Hollander E, Stein DJ, DeCaria C, Cohen LJ, Saoud JB, Islam N, Hwang M. Induction of depersonalization by the serotonin agonist metachlorophenylpiperazine. *Psychiatry Res.* 1995;58:161-4

Simeon D, Guralnik O, Hazlett EA, Spiegel-Cohen J, Hollander E, Buchsbaum MS. Feeling unreal: a PET study of depersonalization disorder. *Am J Psychiatry.* 2000;157:1782-8

Simeon D, Guralnik O, Knutelska M, Yehuda R, Schmeidler J. Basal norepinephrine in depersonalization disorder. *Psych Res.* 2003a;121:93-7

Simeon D, Knutelska M, Nelson D, Guralnik O. Feeling unreal: a depersonalization disorder update of 117 cases. *J Clin Psychiatry.* 2003b;64:990-7

Simeon D, Greenberg J, Nelson D, Schmeidler J, Hollander E. Dissociation and posttraumatic stress 1 year after the World Trade Center disaster: follow-up of a longitudinal survey. *J Clin Psychiatry.* 2005;66:231-7

Smirnov WY. Paroxysmal psychopathological symptoms in patients with brain tumors in the right and left temporal lobes. *Neurosci Behav Physiol.* 1977;8:86-9

Solms M. Freud returns. *Sci Am Mind.* 2006;17:28-33

Southwick SM, Krystal JH, Bremner JD, Morgan CA, Nicolaou AL, Nagy LM, Johnson DR, Heninger GR, Charney DS. Noradrenergic and serotoninergic function in posttraumatic stress disorder. *Arch Gen Psychiatry.* 1997;54:749-58

Spector Person E, Cooper AM, Gabbard GO. *The American Psychiatric Publishing Textbook of Psychoanalysis.* The American Psychiatric Press Pub, Washington, D.C. 2004

Spielberger C. *Manual for the State-Trait Anxiety Inventory (STAI: Form Y).* Consulting Psychologists Press, Palo Alto CA 1983

Steinberg M. *Structured Clinical Interview for DSM-IV Dissociative Disorders-Revised (SCID-D-R).* American Psychiatric Press, Washington, D.C. 1994

Tiihonen J, Kuikka J, Viinamake H, Lehtonen J, Partanen J. Altered cerebral blood flow during hysterical paresthesia. *Biol Psychiat.* 1995;37:134-5

Trimble MR. *Biological psychiatry.* 2nd Edition, John Wiley, Chichester, UK 1996

Trueman D. Depersonalization in a non-clinical population. *J. Psychol.* 1984;116:107-12

Vollenweider FX, Vontobek P, Hell D, Leenders KL. 5-HT modulation of dopamine release in basal ganglia in psylobicin-induced psychosis in man: a PET study with (11C)raclopride. *Neuropsychopharmacol.* 1999;20:424-33

Vuilleumier P. Hysterical conversion and brain function. *Prog Brain Res.* 2005;150:309-29

Vuilleumier P, Chichèrio C, Assal F, Schwarz S, Slosman D, Landis T. Functional neuroanatomical correlates of hysterical sensorimotor loss. *Brain.* 2001;124:1077-90

Walsh SL, Geter-Douglas B, Strain EC. Bigelow GE. Enadoline and butorphanol: evaluation of kappa-agonists on cocaine pharmacodynamics and cocaine self-administration in humans. *J Pharmacol Exp Ther.* 2001;299:147-58

Ward NS, Oakley DA, Frackowiak RSJ, Halligan PM. Differential brain activation during intentionally simulated and subjectively experienced paralysis. *Cogn Neuropsychiatry.* 2003;8:295-312

Wilkes KV. *Real People: Personal Identity Without Thought Experiments.* Oxford: Oxford University Press 1988

Winterer G, Adams CM, Jones DW, Knutson B. Volition to action: an event-related fMRI study. *NeuroImage.* 2002;17:851-8

Wollheim R. *Freud.* 2nd Ed. Harper Collins, London 1991

Yehuda R. Sensitization of the hypothalamic-pituitary-adrenal axis in posttraumatic stress disorder. *Ann N Y Acad Sci.* 1997;821:57-75

Chapter 8

CONCLUSIONS: MIND, MATTER, AND THE CONSCIOUS BRAIN

My brain… That's my second favorite organ!

Woody Allen

As the quintessential human attribute, consciousness has long fascinated philosophers and scientists, not to mention literates and poets. Strangely enough, consciousness has long been shunned by researchers studying the brain and the mind. A century ago William James, the father of American psychology, stated that consciousness is not a thing but a process. The exact nature of this process was to be discovered. However, for many years after James penned "The Principles of Psychology" (1890), consciousness was a taboo concept in American psychology because of the dominance of the behaviorist movement, which focused on external behavior and disallowed any talk of internal mental processes. With the advent of cognitive science in the mid-1950s, it became possible once more for psychologists to consider mental processes as opposed to merely observing behavior. In other words, the rise of cognitive science focused attention on processes inside the head. In spite of these changes, until recently most cognitive scientists ignored consciousness, as did almost all neuroscientists. The problem was felt to be either purely "philosophical" or too elusive to study experimentally. It would not have been easy for a neuroscientist to get a grant to study consciousness, and the mere mention of the "c" word in a scientific report would cause the editor of a neuroscience journal to question the very sanity of the researcher who dared mention it. The prevailing view was that science, which depends on objectivity, could not accommodate something as subjective as consciousness. Only recently an increasing number of neuroscientists, psychologists and philosophers have been rejecting the idea that consciousness cannot be studied and are attempting to delve into its secrets.

In this book we have adopted the clinical perspective of neuropsychiatry to provide an overview of what we know about consciousness and its neural correlates, by assuming that consciousness can not be investigated without keeping in mind both the subject of conscious experience and his brain. We believe that neuroscience can enhance our appreciation of each individual's inner perspective by revealing the neurobiological underpinnings of the complex interplay of structural, chemical, genetic, environmental, developmental, social, and cultural influences on behavior. Specifically, neuropsychiatry enhances intellectual commerce among related clinical and basic disciplines (i.e. psychiatry, neurology, and neuroscience), thus facilitating the translation of scientific advances into clinical and phenomenological descriptions of conscious states.

A dehumanising, reductionistic and mechanical view of humankind is not the obligatory impact of neuroscience on societies; moreover, science has not yet provided an explanation for the nature of subjective experience. Without this, as scientists, we are forced to understand our subjective world as a mechanical distillation of brain function. The genetic programme produces, in the brain, an organ of majestic complexity, but nothing more. Our current science thus dooms us to an existence in which the only meaning is biological, and is in the relationship between humans, and between humans and their environment. The possibility of meaning beyond this is denied, as subjective experience is seen to arise simply from the programming of neuronal networks within the brain. Science certainly accepts the presence of subjective experience, and thus of a personal consciousness. Physicist Erwin Schrödinger commented that without consciousness the activities of creation would be "played out on empty beaches". Consciousness as formulated by science cannot take this any further forward. Science, as yet, has no means of dealing with creativity and subjective experience. This is not to say that looking for the neural correlates of consciousness is futile. On the contrary, at this very early stage of the neurobiological investigation of consciousness, it is undoubtedly wise to give it the best shot possible. Notoriously, science can only analyse those "quality of the world" that appear as third party experience. Therefore, when an explanation for subjective experience is found, then the relationship of conscious experience to the world we live in will have to be rethought.

It appears that not only can our brain-states result in consciousness, but that consciousness has causal efficacy: it can make things happen. Our appreciation of this dates back to more than two millennia ago, when Virgil wrote that "Mens agitat molem" ("mind moves matter", Aeneid, VI, 727). We act on reasons, on knowledge, on hunches, on intuitions that appear to be irreducible to simply biological processes. Indeed, if consciousness did not have such causal efficacy, it is hard to see why it evolved in the first place or why it has come to be such an important part of life. But so put, we are in danger of sliding into Cartesian dualism - that is, of postulating two kinds of substances in the world, physical ones and mental ones - and then having the intractable problem of how they relate. This is a position that most contemporary neurophilosophers and neuroscientists robustly resist. The current orthodoxy believes that all aspects of mind, including its most puzzling attribute – consciousness – are likely to be explainable in a more materialistic way as the behavior of large sets of interacting neurons. The overwhelming question in neurobiology today is the relationship between consciousness and the brain. Everyone agrees that what we know as the continuum of our conscious experiences is closely related to certain aspects of the behavior of the brain, not to the heart, as for instance Aristotle thought. On the current scene, theories concerning the neural substrates of consciousness tend to fall into two broad classes: (1) those who hypothesize that the discharge activity of particular subpopulations of neurons are sufficient to support conscious awareness and to modulate its experiential contents and (2) those who hypothesize that some coherent organization of neural signaling processes, such as well-formed cognitive representations, interneural synchrony, neuronal oscillations, adaptive resonances, or self-regenerating reverberatory patterns, are necessary and sufficient for conscious awareness.

We believe that neuronal-specificity and process-coherence are not necessarily mutually exclusive, since there might well be only particular neural populations that, by virtue of their position within the system, are capable of producing the kinds of organized, self-sustaining activity that coherence theories require. This volume presented a brief overview on what we know about the pathophysiology of consciousness. We have shown that a clinical neuropsychiatry approach leads to a two-dimension model of consciousness, with two separate neuronal network substrates the level of awareness and the specific contents of the conscious states. On the one hand, the level of arousal depends on sustained activity within the reticular formation of the brainstem, the non-specific nuclei of the thalamus, and the fronto-parietal association cortices (with a posteromedial-midfrontal core), which is suspended in sleep, comatose states, artificially-induced anesthesia, and certain epileptic seizures. On the other hand, the specific contents of the conscious states are somewhat related to the limbic structures located in the medial temporal lobe, whose activation supports neural representations that determine the contents or the emotional flavour of our conscious experiences.

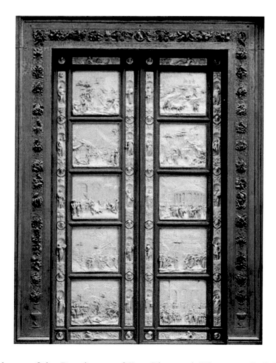

Figure 8.1. The eastern doors of the Baptistery of San Giovanni (Florence, Italy), cast by Renaissance goldsmith, sculptor, architect and author Lorenzo Ghiberti (1378-1455). Impressed by Ghiberti's craftsmanship, Michelangelo Buonarroti (1476-1564), the Italian High Renaissance artist and poet, later called the sculptor's glorious doors the *Gates of Paradise* because he thought they were worthy to stand at the entrance to heaven.

We acknowledge that, at present, it is not possible to provide a more exhaustive account for the multifaceted notion of consciousness and, most importantly, for the neural processes subserving it, the task having to be reserved for future study. However, as a closing remark, we wish to point out that clinical neuropsychiatry will provide one of the most promising avenues for the new field of consciousness studies. As it has been shown in this volume, the time of indulging in the lure of pure poetical representation and philosophical speculation on consciousness has come to an end. It is now mandatory for neuroscientists, psychologists, and philosophers of mind to pursue a great experimental offensive move in order to find the explanatory neurobiological key to open in the next future - who knows? - the "heaven's doors" of human mind (Figure 8.1).

INDEX

A

access, 1, 26, 28, 29, 30, 76
accidents, 132
accounting, 88, 108, 112, 116
accuracy, 66
acetylcholine, 42, 45, 60, 77
acetylcholinesterase, 77, 117
acetylcholinesterase inhibitor, 117
acid, 44, 48, 49, 118
acquisitions, 36
ACTH, 45
action potential, 40, 42, 45
activation, 32, 46, 52, 55, 56, 57, 58, 59, 62, 72, 73,
   82, 89, 92, 100, 102, 110, 122, 133, 135, 136,
   137, 138, 141, 143, 147
adenosine, 45
ADH, 16
adolescence, 126
adrenaline, 48
adults, 58
Africa, 5
age, 5, 40, 74, 79, 82, 88, 97, 105, 106, 107, 109,
   117, 118, 122, 124, 126, 133
ageing, 111, 122, 123
agent, 28, 57, 76, 117
aggregates, 110
aggression, 48
aggressive behavior, 55
aggressiveness, 116
aging, 114, 121, 124
agnosia, 106, 114
agonist, 136, 142
akathisia, 106
akinesia, 114

alcohol, 49, 51, 55, 115
alcohol consumption, 115
alcoholism, 68
alertness, 2, 44, 47, 48, 114, 135
alexia, 106
alienation, 136
allele, 121, 126
alternative, 1, 95
American Psychiatric Association, 105, 122, 132
amnesia, 46, 89, 115, 130, 131, 133, 134, 142
amphetamines, 47, 48
amygdala, 26, 44, 46, 52, 92, 101, 103, 133, 135,
   136, 138
amyloid angiopathy, 110
amyotrophic lateral sclerosis, 110
anatomy, 18, 32, 57, 67, 75, 99, 110, 123, 141
anesthetics, 74, 75, 76, 77, 82
anger, 27, 90, 97
animal models, 87
animals, 26, 75
anterior cingulate cortex, 138, 142
anticholinergic, 77
anticonvulsant, 51
antidepressant, 88
antigen, 53
anti-inflammatory drugs, 109
antioxidant, 117
antipsychotic, 88, 118
anxiety, 73, 97, 106, 108, 130, 132, 136, 141
anxiety disorder, 97, 130, 136, 141
apathy, 106, 108, 115
aphasia, 66, 86, 101, 106, 114, 124
aphonia, 67
aplasia, 123
appetite, 106, 108
apraxia, 66, 106, 108, 114, 115, 116

archeology, 17
arginine, 43
argument, 11
aripiprazole, 118
Aristotle, 146
arousal, 21, 22, 41, 44, 45, 54, 61, 62, 63, 69, 70, 72,
    76, 88, 92, 93, 95, 122, 147
arrest, 131
arteries, 110, 115
arterioles, 110
Artificial Intelligence, 11
aspartate, 48, 125, 140
assessment, viii, 29, 61, 66, 68, 78, 79, 87, 96, 98,
    111, 119, 124, 127, 134, 138
assets, 79
assumptions, 30, 139
asymmetry, 121
ataxia, 114, 115
atherosclerosis, 123
atrophy, 110, 111, 112, 113, 115, 117, 126
attacks, 53, 91, 115, 132
attention, 2, 12, 21, 24, 25, 29, 31, 48, 72, 76, 86, 94,
    95, 96, 97, 101, 105, 113, 114, 115, 118, 121,
    132, 138, 145
attitudes, 12
auditory hallucinations, 18, 48
aura, 89, 90, 91, 92, 99, 101, 102, 115, 133, 139, 141
autobiographical memory, 120, 121
automata, 4
automatisms, 89
autonomy, 111
autopsy, 53
autosomal dominant, 109, 112, 115
availability, 74
awareness, 2, 3, 21, 24, 32, 41, 53, 54, 61, 62, 63,
    64, 65, 66, 67, 69, 70, 72, 73, 76, 85, 87, 89, 90,
    94, 96, 97, 98, 119, 120, 122, 125, 130, 131, 132,
    135, 147
axons, 41, 42

B

Baars, vii, 28, 29, 30, 72, 78, 88, 99, 120, 123
barbiturates, 49, 74
basal forebrain, 41, 43, 117
basal ganglia, 46, 52, 106, 115, 135, 136, 139, 140,
    143
basilar artery, 63, 67
BD, 31, 114
Beck Depression Inventory, 96

behavior, 8, 25, 29, 30, 54, 59, 65, 66, 79, 87, 88, 94,
    95, 102, 120, 145, 146
behavioral change, 100
behavioral problems, 112
behaviorism, 2
benign, 116, 124
benzene, 49
benzodiazepines, 49, 51, 74, 76, 126
beta wave, 41
bicamerality, 3, 5
binding, 24, 48, 49, 51
biological markers, 111
biological processes, 146
birth, 55
bladder, 54
blindness, 135
blocks, 48, 75
blood, 4, 36, 40, 45, 48, 51, 52, 75, 77, 79, 80, 87,
    110, 116, 122, 136
blood flow, 45, 52, 75, 79, 87, 136
blood pressure, 36, 40
blood supply, 122
blood vessels, 110
blood-brain barrier, 77
body image, 132
body schema, 137
body temperature, 48
borderline personality disorder, 133, 136, 139
bradykinesia, 108, 109
brain, 1, 2, 3, 5, 6, 8, 9, 10, 11, 12, 14, 15, 16, 18,
    19, 20, 21, 23, 24, 25, 26, 27, 28, 29, 30, 31, 32,
    35, 36, 40, 41, 46, 47, 52, 55, 56, 57, 61, 62, 63,
    64, 66, 68, 69, 70, 71, 72, 73, 74, 75, 76, 77, 78,
    79, 80, 81, 83, 87, 89, 91, 92, 99, 100, 101, 102,
    106, 107, 111, 112, 115, 116, 119, 121, 122, 123,
    125, 126, 127, 132, 134, 136, 137, 139, 143, 145,
    146
brain activity, 11, 63, 101, 127
brain damage, 27, 61, 63, 64, 72, 80
brain imaging techniques, 75, 122, 134
brain stem, 62, 63, 78
brain structure, 21, 27, 30, 41, 46, 102, 126
brain tumor, 111, 143
brainstem, 21, 27, 29, 41, 42, 43, 44, 45, 46, 47, 56,
    57, 60, 61, 62, 63, 64, 65, 66, 67, 69, 71, 72, 76,
    87, 88, 93, 106, 114, 147
brainstem nuclei, 114
breakdown, 3, 56
breathing, 53

C

caffeine, 47
calcium, 42
cannabinoids, 135, 136
capillary, 45
capsule, 115
carbon, 122
carbon monoxide, 122
caregivers, 117
carotid arteries, 7
Cartesian cut, 5, 6, 16
cast, 147
cataplexy, 53
catastrophes, 5
catatonia, 68, 132
catatonic, 67, 68
catatonic schizophrenia, 67
causal relationship, 20
causation, 10
CE, 32, 102, 125, 139
cell, 49, 110, 117
cell body, 110
cell membranes, 117
central nervous system, 21, 29, 74, 75, 76, 77, 79, 82, 134
central pontine myelinolysis, 67
cerebellum, 26, 93
cerebral arteries, 122
cerebral blood flow, 52, 56, 75, 76, 80, 81, 83, 87, 121, 135, 141, 143
cerebral cortex, 23, 27, 31, 46, 47, 48, 64, 68, 75, 102, 109, 110, 122, 142
cerebral hemisphere, 22, 72
cerebral hypoxia, 64
cerebral metabolism, 71, 72, 75, 77, 83
cerebrospinal fluid, 53, 58, 111, 116, 124
cerebrovascular disease, 63, 111
certainty, 64
C-fibres, 13
Chalmers, vii, 2, 8, 9, 16, 20, 30, 94, 99
channels, 12, 42, 49
chaos, 5
Charles Darwin, 9
childhood, 86, 87, 103, 126, 137
childhood sexual abuse, 137
children, 54, 55, 64, 78, 82
China, 5
chloral, 49
cholesterol, 109, 114, 123

cholinergic neurons, 42, 44, 45, 58, 109, 110
cholinesterase, 117
cholinesterase inhibitors, 117
chorea, 114
chromosome, 109, 113
chronic pain, 141
circadian oscillator, 45
circadian rhythm, 43, 45, 53, 59
circadian rhythm sleep disorders, 53
circadian rhythmicity, 43, 45
circadian rhythms, 43, 59
circulation, 63, 65
citalopram, 118
classes, 21, 135, 146
classification, 17, 56, 66, 86, 94, 100, 101, 106, 107, 130
clinical assessment, 61, 69, 122, 123
clinical examination, 110
clinical syndrome, 30, 65, 106, 116
closure, 14, 65, 68
CNS, 47, 49, 51, 140, 142
cocaine, 55, 143
codes, 115
coding, 56
cognition, 6, 117, 120, 138, 142
cognitive abilities, 67
cognitive capacities, 15
cognitive deficit, 105, 106, 119, 120, 124
cognitive deficits, 105, 120
cognitive domains, 116, 120
cognitive dysfunction, 119
cognitive function, 2, 20, 66, 105, 111, 120
cognitive impairment, 106, 113, 115, 116, 117, 118, 120, 126
cognitive process, 27, 30, 66, 73, 140
cognitive processing, 66, 73
cognitive profile, 114
cognitive psychology, 8
cognitive representations, 147
cognitive science, 16, 145
cognitive slowing, 114
cognitive system, 8
cognitive tasks, 89
coherence, 25, 129, 147
Colin McGinn, vii, 14
collaboration, 22
coma, 2, 18, 20, 32, 49, 61, 62, 63, 64, 65, 68, 69, 71, 73, 76, 80, 81, 82, 83, 88, 89
combustibility, 12
commerce, 146

common symptoms, 53

communication, 58, 65, 67, 113

comorbidity, 111

competence, 15

competition, 11, 26, 28

complex behaviors, 102

complex interactions, 56

complex partial seizure, 86, 89, 92, 93, 95, 98, 100, 103

complexity, 27, 33, 146

complications, 108

components, 28, 69, 76, 90, 92, 98, 126, 132, 136, 137

comprehension, 65, 108, 113

computed tomography, 87

computer simulations, 25

computing, 18

concentration, 36, 48, 74

conception, 6

concussion, 64

conductor, 56

confidence, 48

conflict, 134

confusion, 68, 129, 130

Congress, 67, 77

connectivity, 56, 58, 72, 75, 80, 81, 83, 88, 122, 124, 137

conscious activity, 6

conscious awareness, 17, 21, 32, 41, 75, 100, 147

conscious experiences, 1, 8, 29, 36, 97, 99, 146, 147

conscious knowledge, 11

conscious perception, 27, 114

consciousness, vii, viii, 1, 2, 3, 4, 5, 6, 8, 9, 10, 11, 12, 14, 15, 16, 17, 18, 19, 20, 21, 22, 23, 24, 25, 26, 27, 28, 29, 30, 31, 32, 33, 35, 46, 52, 53, 54, 56, 57, 60, 61, 62, 63, 64, 65, 66, 67, 68, 70, 71, 72, 73, 74, 75, 76, 77, 78, 81, 82, 83, 85, 86, 87, 88, 89, 90, 91, 92, 93, 94, 95, 96, 97, 98, 99, 101, 102, 103, 106, 108, 111, 112, 118, 119, 120, 121, 123, 126, 127, 129, 130, 134, 138, 139, 145, 146, 147, 148

consensus, 19, 65, 125, 129

conservation, 23, 112

consolidation, 55, 57, 59, 60

construction, 25, 30

consultants, 81

continuity, 4, 11, 25, 129

control, 8, 12, 29, 43, 45, 46, 58, 59, 64, 75, 81, 82, 95, 96, 97, 99, 114, 133, 135

conversion, 130, 134, 138, 139, 140, 141, 143

conversion disorder, 130, 134, 135, 138, 139, 141

correlation, 20, 24, 71, 101, 119

correlations, 14, 20, 21, 62, 98, 99, 123

cortex, 2, 21, 23, 24, 26, 27, 29, 32, 42, 44, 46, 52, 62, 63, 72, 73, 83, 87, 88, 89, 93, 102, 110, 121, 122, 125, 135, 137, 138, 139

corticobasal degeneration, 114

coupling, 58, 88

covering, 131

cranial nerve, 64, 66

creativity, 23, 146

criticism, 5, 8

crying, 66

cues, 43

cultural influence, 29, 146

culture, 4, 30

cuneiform, 4

cycles, 40, 44, 45, 64, 65, 68

cytokines, 45, 52

D

daily living, 117

danger, 12, 142, 146

Daniel Dennett, vii, 11

Darwin's theory, 9

Darwinism, 26, 28

death, 7, 35, 48, 49, 61, 63, 70, 71, 79, 81, 83, 107, 112, 114, 119, 132

decay, 105

decisions, 4, 5

declarative knowledge, 57

declarative memory, 56, 59, 60

deficiency, 59, 107

deficit, 48, 105, 107, 108, 113, 119, 127, 138

definition, 2, 9, 28, 30, 65, 78, 79, 82, 115, 129, 130

degenerate, 110

degenerative dementia, 106, 118, 119

delirium, 48, 105, 130, 132

delivery, 109

delta wave, 55

delusion, 107

delusions, 68, 114

dementia, 105, 106, 107, 108, 109, 110, 111, 112, 113, 114, 115, 116, 117, 118, 120, 121, 122, 123, 124, 125, 126, 127

demographic characteristics, 124

density, 56, 110

Department of Health and Human Services, 125

dependent variable, 74

depersonalization, 130, 132, 135, 136, 137, 138, 140, 141, 142

depolarization, 43, 60

deposits, 109, 110

depression, 48, 49, 51, 63, 67, 77, 78, 83, 90, 99, 106, 108, 115, 118, 130, 132

deprivation, 48, 54

derivatives, 49

desire, 23

desires, 9

destruction, 41, 53

detachment, 132, 137

detection, 2, 110

developmental psychopathology, 140

deviation, 70

diabetes, 109, 114

diabetes mellitus, 109

diagnostic criteria, 65, 66, 79, 82, 112, 125, 126

differential diagnosis, 32, 103, 110, 111, 113, 114, 139

differentiation, 87, 106

digestion, 1

disability, 115

disaster, 130, 142

discharges, 42, 54, 87, 92, 95, 100, 101

discipline, 29

discomfort, 91

discourse, 12

disease progression, 111, 113

disinhibition, 106

disorder, ix, 48, 53, 54, 57, 58, 59, 99, 106, 129, 132, 133, 134, 135, 136, 137, 138, 139, 140, 141, 142, 143

dissatisfaction, 86

dissociation, 55, 92, 130, 131, 132, 133, 136, 139, 140, 141

dissociative disorders, 129, 130, 134, 138

dissociative fugue, 130

dissociative identity disorder, 130, 133, 139

distillation, 146

distribution, 29, 89, 113

doctors, 117

dogs, 53

dominance, 29, 145

doors, 147, 148

dopamine, 47, 48, 136, 143

dorsolateral prefrontal cortex, 46, 52, 121, 138

dosing, 74

Down syndrome, 109

draft, 11

dream, 40, 46, 47, 53, 55, 57, 60, 91, 96, 132

dreaming, 36, 40, 41, 46, 50, 55, 58, 59, 75, 82

drug abuse, 48, 129

drug action, 74

drug interaction, 47

drugs, 41, 47, 49, 50, 73, 74, 75, 76, 77, 132

DSM, 105, 118, 122, 129, 130, 132, 134, 143

DSM-IV, 105, 118, 122, 129, 130, 132, 134, 143

dualism, 2, 5, 8, 9, 10, 22, 23, 146

duration, 6, 36, 40, 45, 48, 49, 50, 51, 97

dysarthria, 114

dysphagia, 115

E

ears, 6

earth, 85

eating, 108

ECM, 140

Education, 28

educational process, 120

EEG, 32, 36, 37, 38, 39, 40, 41, 42, 49, 55, 56, 59, 73, 74, 75, 82, 86, 87, 88, 93, 97, 101, 102, 103, 110, 134

EEG patterns, 41, 42

ego, 119, 121, 139

Egypt, 5

elderly, 40, 106, 107, 110, 122

electric current, 88

electrodes, 88, 91

electron, 116

electron microscopy, 116

emergence, 11, 25

EMG, 36

emission, 57, 77, 79, 87, 111, 112

emotion, 27, 29, 31, 102, 123, 126

emotional disorder, 134

emotional experience, 90, 95, 97, 121

emotional responses, 28

emotional stimuli, 53, 66

emotionality, 46

emotions, 6, 9, 12, 21, 27, 97, 103, 121, 138, 140

encephalitis, 67, 117

encephalopathy, 82, 107, 116

endocrine, 45

energy, 2, 23

enlargement, 116

entorhinal cortex, 122

environment, 2, 21, 41, 42, 52, 54, 61, 62, 64, 65, 66, 69, 72, 85, 89, 94, 95, 120, 129, 130, 146 environmental awareness, 65, 66

environmental influences, 29

environmental stimuli, 27, 66

enzymes, 109

epidemiology, 132

epidermoid cyst, 79

epilepsy, 12, 17, 21, 54, 85, 86, 87, 88, 90, 91, 94, 95, 98, 99, 100, 101, 102, 103, 130, 132, 134, 137, 139, 140, 141

epileptic seizures, 17, 48, 58, 85, 86, 88, 89, 91, 98, 100, 101, 103, 139, 147

episodic memory, 78, 108, 131

estrangement, 132

ethanol, 51

ethyl alcohol, 51

etiology, xi, 67, 112, 122

Euclidean space, 16

euphoria, 48, 90, 106

evoked potential, 73, 135, 140

evolution, 5, 9, 111, 112, 117, 126, 134, 140

evolutionary process, 3

examinations, 113

excitability, 44, 48

excitation, 23, 48

exclusion, 112, 135

executive function, 81, 114, 115

executive functions, 81, 114

exercise, 29

exposure, 43

extensor, 69

external environment, 11, 41, 43, 94

eye movement, 36, 40, 43, 50, 59, 66, 67

eyes, 6, 40, 54, 63, 64, 69, 83, 105

F

failure, 62, 69, 105, 108

fatigue, 35, 48, 129

fear, 73, 90, 97, 100, 102

feedback, 26, 45, 76

feelings, 9, 12, 21, 27, 73, 90, 91, 94, 132, 138

feet, 116

fever, 54

fibers, 29, 44

fibroblasts, 111

fixation, 66

flame, 17

flashbacks, 97

flexibility, 28, 68

fluid, 126

fluoxetine, 118

focal seizure, 87, 92, 93, 98, 101

focusing, 54, 94

forebrain, 41, 46, 52, 60, 109, 110

forgetting, 47, 113, 131

fractures, 130

fragmentation, 36, 129

France, iii

free will, 15, 24, 120, 126

freedom, 23

frontal cortex, 50, 135

frontal lobe, 24, 54, 93, 100, 106, 119, 121, 127

frontotemporal dementia, 110, 119, 123, 124, 125

frontotemporal lobar degeneration, 106

frustration, 73

fugue, ix, 131

functional activation, 21

functional imaging, 29, 52, 72, 80, 92, 139

functional MRI, 78, 112, 124, 141

G

gait, 115, 116

ganglion, 43

gender, 74, 82

gene, 45, 53, 58, 109, 115

general anesthesia, 88, 89

general knowledge, 131

generalization, 25

generalized amnesia, 131

generalized seizures, 87, 88, 98

generalized tonic-clonic seizure, 86, 87

generation, 42, 54, 57, 59, 71, 107, 117

genes, 116

genetics, 29, 59, 109

genotype, 109

gestures, 28

ghost, 2

gift, 31

gland, 6, 52

glass, 10

glucose, 52, 55, 72, 77, 78, 79, 80, 81, 82, 83, 122

glutamate, 44, 51, 135

goal-oriented behaviour, 122

God, 14

government, iv

grading, 111

grey matter, 62, 71

groups, 26, 42, 57, 113, 118, 119, 137

growth, 29, 36, 44, 64

growth factor, 45
growth hormone, 44
guidance, 83
guidelines, 79, 125
guilt, 90
guilty, 54

H

hallucinations, 5, 68, 86, 89, 90, 91, 97, 106, 113, 114
happiness, 97
HE, 141
head injury, 64, 78, 79, 80
head trauma, 71, 78
headache, 48
health, 140
heart disease, 109, 114
heart rate, 40, 65, 70
heat, 6, 14, 42
hemiparesis, 63
hemisphere, 5, 62, 113, 137
hemorrhage, 73, 116
hepatotoxicity, 117
heterogeneity, 83, 124
heterophenomenology, 11
hieratic, 4
hieroglyphics, 4
hippocampus, 26, 44, 55, 110, 115, 121, 126, 135, 136
HLA, 53, 58
homunculi, 12
Honda, 58
hormone, 44, 52
HPA axis, 136
human actions, 4
human behavior, 29, 30
human brain, xi, 5, 11, 31, 32, 75, 80, 102
human cerebral cortex, 78
human experience, 30, 92
hydrocephalus, 107, 116, 123, 124
hyperactivity, 48
hyperphosphorylated tau protein, 110
hypertension, 48, 109, 114
hypnagogic hallucinations, 53
hypnosis, 5, 12, 36, 131, 133, 140
hypochondriasis, 140
hypothalamus, 26, 41, 42, 43, 44, 45, 48, 49, 52, 62
hypothermia, 63

hypothesis, 3, 4, 5, 16, 24, 25, 27, 30, 31, 46, 47, 52, 55, 57, 75, 76, 80, 87, 89, 93, 122, 124, 136, 138
hypoxia, 122

I

ICD, 129, 130
identification, 20, 30, 59, 98, 107
identity, ix, 119, 129, 130, 131, 133
idiopathic, 30, 116
idiosyncratic, 101
Iliad, 4, 5
illusion, 89
illusions, 6, 89, 97
imagery, 25, 46, 53, 137, 141
imaging, 57, 71, 73, 75, 77, 80, 81, 87, 98, 111, 115, 121, 123, 135, 136
imbalances, 68
Immanuel Kant, 15
immunization, 117, 125
impairments, 53, 76, 114, 116, 132
in situ, 27
in vitro, 57, 58, 77, 83
in vivo, 77
inattention, 86
incidence, 88, 106, 114
inclusion, 86
India, 5
induction, 135, 136
inertia, 106
infants, 36
infarction, 63, 73
inferences, 61
infinite, 14
inflammation, 117, 123
information processing, 87, 102
ingestion, 48, 51
inhibition, 35, 41, 43, 44, 54, 58, 93, 136, 137, 138
inhibitor, 51, 77, 117
initiation, 44, 138
input, 29, 48, 137
insight, 4, 30, 119, 120, 127, 132
insomnia, 49
insulin, 45
integration, 25, 26, 55, 60, 68, 130, 132, 137
integrity, 21, 66, 72, 121
intelligence, 15, 105
intentions, 21
interaction, 6, 7, 11, 21, 23, 25, 26, 27, 31, 46, 69, 80, 138

interactions, 75, 77, 88, 135, 137
interface, 138, 142
interference, 28
internal clock, 43
interneurons, 81
interpersonal relations, 29
interpersonal relationships, 29
interpretation, 9, 24, 30, 52, 87, 139
intervention, 127
intoxication, 55, 63
intracranial pressure, 116
introspection, 3, 14, 15, 119
intrusions, 53
ipsilateral, 93
irritability, 106, 108, 116
ischemia, 115
Islam, 142
isolation, 89, 90
Italy, 147

J

Jaynes, 3, 4, 5, 16, 17
Jaynes' theory, 3
John Searle, vii, 10, 94
joints, 4
judgment, 65, 112
justification, 66

L

language, 3, 4, 25, 26, 27, 30, 65, 66, 72, 105, 108, 113, 120
language skills, 108
latency, 48, 49, 50, 51
laterality, 137
laughing, 55, 66
learning, 4, 25, 57, 60
left hemisphere, 5, 137
leptomeninges, 110
lesions, 21, 30, 62, 63, 68, 71, 73, 76, 106, 110, 115, 116, 121, 137
lifetime, 55
light cycle, 52
limbic system, 26, 32, 49, 100, 137
limitation, 65, 69
linkage, 109
lipid metabolism, 109
lipid peroxidation, 117

liquidity, 10
liver, 48
localization, 6, 101, 142
location, 49, 66, 115
locus, 12, 42, 44, 48, 59
logical reasoning, 6
loss of consciousness, 35, 75, 76, 79, 86, 87, 88, 93, 100, 101, 103, 114, 117, 120
LSD, 136

M

machinery, 22
magnetic resonance, 52, 58, 62, 80, 88, 106, 141
magnetic resonance imaging, 52, 58, 62, 80, 88, 106
magnetism, 1
major depression, 88
malingering, 141
management, 61, 79, 83, 117, 123, 126
manipulation, 70, 75
mapping, 87, 126
marijuana, 135
materialism, 13, 22
maturation, 55, 121
meanings, 2
measurement, 58, 74
measures, 21, 120, 122
median, 42, 45
mediation, 30
melatonin, 43, 45, 52
memory, 2, 25, 26, 55, 60, 72, 86, 90, 105, 106, 107, 108, 113, 114, 116, 120, 121, 129, 130, 131, 132, 135, 137, 141
memory loss, 108, 116, 131
memory performance, 117
memory processes, 60
men, 5
mental activity, 4, 12, 36
mental disorder, 122
mental impairment, 116
mental life, 4
mental processes, 145
mental representation, 2
mental state, 2, 9, 12, 13, 14, 20, 90, 98, 101
mental states, 2, 9, 12, 13, 14, 20, 98, 101
Mesoamerica, 5
messages, 28
metabolic dysfunction, 72
metabolism, 71, 72, 73, 75, 77, 78, 79, 80, 82, 83, 87, 120, 122

metacognition, 119
metaphor, 3, 9, 56
mice, 117
microscopy, 116
microstructure, 23
midbrain, 41, 42, 49, 52, 73, 79
migraine, 130
mild cognitive impairment, 116, 122
military, 133
mind-body, 2, 10, 13, 16
mind-body problem, 2, 10, 13, 16
minority, 115
model system, 27
models, 3, 28
modules, 56
molecular biology, 29, 109
molecules, 10, 24
mood, 97, 111, 117, 120, 141
mood disorder, 111, 117
morning, 54
morphology, 103
motion, 14, 23, 46, 67, 96
motivation, 29, 120
motor activity, 43, 44, 48
motor control, 135, 142
motor neurons, 43
motor system, 66
moulding, 22
movement, 53, 54, 67, 70, 94, 114, 138, 145
movement disorders, 53, 114
MRI, 52, 62, 73, 80, 82, 88, 103, 111, 112, 122, 126, 137
multi-infarct dementia, 115
multiple personality, 130, 133
multiple personality disorder, 130, 133
multiple sclerosis, 63
muscle cells, 116
muscle relaxant, 49, 51
muscles, 40, 54
music, 27, 56, 89, 91
mutation, 53, 58, 59, 109, 113, 115, 117
mutations, 29, 107
Mycenaean, 4
myocardial infarction, 48
myoclonus, 109

N

narcolepsy, 48, 53, 55, 58, 59, 60
narratives, 11, 12

natural selection, 9, 15
negative emotions, 73
neocortex, 23, 55, 87, 92, 107
neonates, 55
neoplasia, 107
nerve, 24, 63, 110
nerve cells, 24
nerves, 18
nervous system, 28, 29, 75
network, 24, 52, 72, 75, 76, 80, 83, 87, 93, 99, 124, 138, 147
neural mechanisms, 98, 122
neural network, 2, 12, 29, 52, 73, 75, 76, 77, 89, 121
neural networks, 2, 12, 75, 121
neural systems, 134
neurobiology, 8, 10, 30, 47, 57, 59, 75, 81, 138, 141, 146
neurodegenerative disorders, 106
neurofibrillary tangles, 106, 107, 110
neurofilament, 114
neuroimaging, 20, 21, 45, 46, 52, 61, 62, 65, 75, 76, 81, 85, 102, 111, 137
neuroimaging techniques, 20, 52, 75
neurological condition, 130
neurological deficit, 115, 135
neurological disability, 78
neurological disease, 131
neurological disorder, 55, 64, 111
neurologist, 26, 27, 89
neuronal death, 72
neuronal systems, 57
neurons, 23, 24, 25, 26, 41, 42, 43, 44, 45, 48, 49, 52, 56, 57, 59, 60, 75, 81, 82, 83, 110, 112, 117, 146
neuropharmacology, 56
neurophysiology, 2, 7, 47, 58
neuroprotective, 117
neuropsychiatry, 29, 30, 31, 32, 145, 147, 148
neuropsychological tests, 110, 112
neuropsychology, 29
neuroscience, 8, 9, 20, 29, 30, 31, 57, 59, 77, 123, 139, 145, 146
neuroses, 141
neurosurgery, 31, 100
neurotransmission, 22, 45, 117, 135
neurotransmitter, 23, 30, 42, 109, 136
neurotransmitters, 44, 77
nightmares, 50
nitrous oxide, 80
NMDA receptors, 135, 136

Nobel Prize, 25, 47
noise, 72
non-clinical population, 143
nonconscious, 4, 5
norepinephrine, 142
normal aging, 122
normal pressure hydrocephalus, 111, 123
nuclei, 21, 29, 42, 43, 44, 45, 46, 56, 62, 72, 73, 76, 87, 122, 126, 147
nucleus, 40, 41, 42, 44, 52, 57, 59, 76, 109, 110, 119, 135
nymph, 54

O

objectivity, 145
observations, 89
obsessive-compulsive disorder, 137
obstructive sleep apnoea, 54
occipital cortex, 40, 136
occipital lobe, 93, 110, 137
occipital regions, 114
occlusion, 67
ocular movements, 36, 67
oculomotor, 43, 81
Odyssey, 4
olanzapine, 118
old age, 109
older adults, 123
opioids, 74
optic nerve, 2, 43
organ, 6, 19, 145, 146
organic disease, 68
organism, 25, 26, 27
organization, 11, 12, 28, 40, 121, 139, 147
orientation, 69, 112
oscillation, 57
outpatients, 118
output, 29, 44, 45, 113
overpopulation, 5
oxygen, 52, 72, 80
oxygen consumption, 52, 80

P

pain, 1, 8, 9, 13, 14, 54, 69, 70, 81, 91, 126, 134
panic disorder, 130
paradigm shift, 5
parallelism, 120

paralysis, 54, 66, 135, 140, 141, 143
parameter, 83, 124
parietal cortex, 73, 76, 93, 120, 122
parietal lobe, 52, 111, 121
parkinsonism, 113, 114
paroxetine, 118
partial seizure, 85, 86, 93, 100, 102, 103, 133
passive, 41, 68
pathogenesis, 113, 133
pathologic diagnosis, 125
pathology, xi, 67, 113, 115, 116, 122, 126
pathophysiology, 29, 147
pathways, 2, 66, 78, 117, 122
patient care, 74
Paul Churchland, vii, 12
peptides, 45, 59
perception, 2, 4, 8, 14, 23, 27, 46, 61, 86, 129, 130, 132, 137, 138
perceptions, 1, 9, 12, 23, 25, 120, 137, 138, 139
perfusion, 71, 82, 103, 112
peritoneum, 80
permit, 75
personal identity, 24
personal life, 90
personality, 106, 108, 112, 117, 131, 133
personality disorder, 108
personality traits, 131
PET, 52, 56, 71, 72, 73, 76, 77, 78, 80, 81, 102, 112, 135, 136, 137, 142, 143
PET scan, 71, 73, 81
pharmacokinetics, 74, 79, 82
pharmacology, 57
pharmacotherapy, 88
phenomenology, 85, 126, 132
phenotype, 113, 114, 117
philosophers, 2, 3, 15, 16, 119, 145, 148
photosynthesis, 1
physical properties, 8, 9
physics, 8, 16, 23
physiology, 36, 59
pilot study, 142
pineal gland, 1, 6, 7, 44, 45, 52
placebo, 136
planning, 138
plasma, 74
plasticity, 56
Plato, 105
pleasure, 90, 91, 97
PM, 16, 80, 101, 126, 139, 143
pneumonia, 96

pons, 40, 41, 42, 45, 52, 54, 63, 67, 115
poor, 105, 115
population, 56, 74, 118
positive correlation, 97
positron, 52, 56, 78, 79, 80, 81, 82, 83, 102, 135
positron emission tomography, 52, 56, 78, 80, 81, 82, 83, 102, 135
posterior cortex, 137
posttraumatic stress, 136, 140, 141, 142, 143
post-traumatic stress disorder, 130
power, 3, 8, 53, 74
prefrontal cortex, 27, 44, 52, 121, 137, 138, 141
president, 81
pressure, 40, 70, 107, 116
primary visual cortex, 24, 31
primate, 140
privacy, 13
probability, 23, 110
problem solving, 108
production, 92, 99, 109, 130
prognosis, xi, 61
program, 11, 117
programming, 57, 146
prolactin, 45
promoter, 48
protective factors, 109
proteins, 110, 114, 123
protocol, 98
pseudobulbar palsy, 115
psychiatric disorders, 30, 67, 88, 130
psychiatric illness, 68
psychiatric patients, 132, 136
psychiatrist, 105, 107, 139
psychoanalysis, 47, 139
psychoanalytic theories, 47
psychobiology, 129
psychological functions, 55
psychological phenomena, 12, 138
psychological stress, 54, 134
psychologist, 3
psychology, 2, 6, 8, 12, 145
psychopathology, 97, 102, 130, 139, 141
psychosis, 48, 118, 143
psychostimulants, 47
ptosis, 81
PTSD, 130, 131, 136, 137, 141
pumps, 74
PVS, 65
pyramidal cells, 24
pyrimidine, 49

Q

qualia, 9, 11, 17, 92, 94, 98, 99, 100, 101
quetiapine, 118

R

race, 48
radio, 92
rain, 72
range, 20, 24, 28, 43, 71, 72, 74, 88, 93, 97, 106, 129, 130
rapid eye movement sleep, 58, 59
ratings, 119
reading, 22, 113
reality, 2, 6, 17, 46, 132, 138
reasoning, 4, 106
recall, 21, 89, 90, 92, 113, 131
recalling, 92
receptor agonist, 135, 136
receptor sites, 49
receptors, 43, 44, 49, 51, 136
recognition, 2, 70, 85, 89, 127
recollection, 89
reconcile, 1
recovery, 61, 64, 65, 67, 69, 78, 81, 115, 131
reduction, 16, 41, 48, 49, 71, 72, 110, 121, 125
reductionism, 22
redundancy, 25
reflection, 118, 119
reflexes, 63, 64, 68, 69, 78, 112
regulation, 27, 53, 65, 76, 102
rehabilitation, 78
relationship, 2, 3, 5, 10, 15, 20, 21, 26, 35, 36, 54, 55, 66, 78, 85, 86, 95, 118, 127, 139, 146
relationships, 10, 30, 47, 74
relativity, 15, 16
relevance, 53, 81, 111, 133, 142
reliability, 86
religious beliefs, 23
REM, 36, 37, 38, 39, 40, 41, 42, 43, 44, 45, 46, 48, 49, 50, 51, 52, 53, 54, 55, 56, 57, 58, 59, 114
René Descartes, 5, 18
reprocessing, 60
reproduction, 1, 92
resolution, 88
respiration, 65
respiratory, 40, 49, 51
responsiveness, 3, 21, 65, 66, 86, 89, 93, 95, 96, 97

reticular activating system, 43, 46, 47, 49, 62, 63, 76
retina, 2
returns, 143
rhythm, 36, 50, 56, 57
rhythmicity, 45, 58
rhythms, 36, 37, 43, 57, 75
right hemisphere, 5, 121
rigidity, 79, 109, 114, 115
risk, 47, 109, 114, 122, 127
risk factors, 109, 114, 127
risperidone, 118

S

sadness, 90, 97
salts, 110
saturation, 36
schizophrenia, 5, 88, 130, 133, 135
scientific community, 9
scientific understanding, 3
sclerosis, 93, 103, 123
scores, 97, 118, 119, 132, 137
search, 2, 16, 31, 80, 92, 99
secrete, 43
secretion, 45
sedative, 49, 74
seizure, 85, 87, 88, 89, 91, 92, 93, 94, 95, 96, 97, 98, 99, 101, 102, 132
seizures, 32, 49, 54, 85, 86, 87, 88, 89, 91, 92, 93, 94, 95, 97, 98, 99, 100, 101, 102, 103, 109, 132, 134, 139
selecting, 22
selectionist principles, 26
selective attention, 95
selective serotonin reuptake inhibitor, 118
selectivity, 25
self-awareness, 25, 73, 120, 122
self-consciousness, 2, 19, 105, 120, 121, 134
self-knowledge, 2
self-reflection, 120, 121, 122
self-regulation, 138
self-understanding, 19
semantic memory, 120, 131
semantics, 26
senescence, 116
senile dementia, 107
senile plaques, 109
sensation, 4, 29, 43, 64, 90, 91, 101, 132, 137
sensations, 1, 6, 8, 9, 21, 25, 27, 89, 101
sensitization, 136

sensory data, 121
sensory systems, 89
series, 11, 15, 27, 65, 113, 130
serotonin, 42, 52, 136, 142
sertraline, 118
serum, 111
severity, 69, 111, 119, 120, 135
sex, 109
sexual abuse, 133
sexual behaviour, 106
shape, 25, 97
short-term memory, 27
side effects, 48, 118
sign, 63, 66, 114, 116
signalling, 75
signals, 27, 45, 65, 135
signs, 61, 63, 64, 65, 68, 73, 106, 108, 112, 113, 114, 115, 117, 119, 130
silver, 110
sites, 49, 75, 136
skeletal muscle, 53
skills, 4, 46, 105
skin, 80, 136
sleep disorders, 36, 47, 53, 56, 114
sleep paralysis, 53, 54
sleep spindle, 37, 41, 42
sleep stage, 40, 52, 58
sleep walking, 54
sleeping pills, 57
smoke, 114
smoking, 109
smooth muscle, 115
smooth muscle cells, 115
social cognition, 59
social institutions, 23
social life, 111
social phobia, 136
society, 28, 31
software, 5, 17
somatization, 134, 140
somatization disorder, 134
somatosensory, 135, 137, 138, 141
somnolence, 41, 60
sounds, 6, 69
spatial information, 15
spatial location, 6
species, 9, 26, 27
specificity, 147
spectrum, 3, 8, 20
speculation, 121, 148

speech, 21, 66, 67, 69, 94, 113
speed, 28, 48, 63
spinal cord, 62
spindle, 42
spine, 79
stages, 36, 37, 40, 41, 45, 48, 49, 50, 51, 52, 54, 56, 61, 64, 65, 68, 108, 112
standards, 41, 88
status epilepticus, 22, 94, 95
stimulus, 69, 121
storage, 47, 55
strategies, 117
stream of consciousness, 32, 102
streams, 95
stress, 5, 54, 73, 129, 135, 136
striatum, 44, 135, 136
stroke, 48, 114
stupor, 2, 18, 32, 67, 82
subcortical infarcts, 115
subcortical structures, 87, 93, 98, 102
subgroups, 53
subjective experience, 2, 8, 11, 20, 21, 22, 29, 30, 87, 94, 95, 96, 97, 138, 146
subjectivity, 2, 4, 25
substrates, 21, 23, 86, 100, 146, 147
subtraction, 32, 101
suffering, 63, 65, 68, 91, 95, 120
supernatural, 19
supply, 25
suppression, 80
suprachiasmatic nucleus, 43, 58
survivors, 64, 71
swelling, 112
symbols, 5, 11
symptom, 131
symptoms, 47, 48, 53, 86, 90, 92, 93, 95, 97, 101, 106, 108, 113, 114, 115, 116, 117, 119, 123, 126, 129, 130, 132, 134, 135, 136, 138, 139, 143
synapse, 10
synaptic transmission, 75
synchronization, 42, 52, 57
syndrome, 50, 66, 67, 68, 73, 78, 79, 80, 81, 82, 106, 107, 112, 114, 115, 116, 123, 132, 133, 136, 140
synergistic effect, 74
synthesis, 46, 57, 121, 126
systems, 2, 12, 23, 25, 26, 31, 46, 62, 69, 83, 109, 117

T

tachycardia, 48
tangles, 107, 110
targets, 21, 73
tau, 110, 113, 117
tautological, 2
teeth, 105
temperature, 42, 45
temporal lobe, viii, 21, 32, 46, 54, 89, 91, 92, 93, 95, 96, 98, 99, 100, 101, 102, 103, 110, 111, 112, 133, 137, 143, 147
temporal lobe epilepsy, viii, 32, 54, 89, 92, 96, 99, 100, 101, 102, 103
tendon, 64
textbooks, xi, 2
thalamocortical pathways, 122
thalamocortical system, 25, 101
thalamus, 24, 26, 27, 29, 42, 44, 45, 48, 49, 52, 60, 62, 71, 75, 76, 77, 88, 93, 99, 106, 115, 122, 135, 136, 138, 147
theory, 1, 3, 5, 9, 12, 15, 16, 22, 23, 24, 25, 26, 27, 28, 30, 31, 41, 46, 53, 60, 77, 82, 99, 101, 141
therapeutic agents, 30
therapeutics, 124
therapy, 88, 100, 106, 117, 142
theta waves, 41
thinking, 4, 6, 23, 106, 120, 142
Thomas Henry Huxley, 9
Thomas Nagel, 15
threshold, 54, 97
thrombosis, 63
TID, 122
time, 2, 4, 7, 9, 10, 11, 24, 26, 28, 35, 41, 42, 43, 46, 48, 50, 51, 61, 65, 77, 78, 96, 97, 115, 117, 121, 131, 132, 148
tissue, 9, 53, 93, 107
tonic, 56, 87, 98
traffic, 94
traits, 76, 130
transducer, 52
transection, 56
transient ischemic attack, 115
transition, 3, 4, 36, 54, 65, 76, 130
transitions, 41
translation, 13, 146
transmission, 77, 112
transparency, 10
trauma, 71, 72, 80, 131, 133
traumatic brain injury, 67, 78, 79, 80, 126, 131

tremor, 48, 114, 134
trend, 120
trial, 60, 117, 139
trisomy, 109
trisomy 21, 109
tryptophan, 52
tumor, 73
tumours, 67

U

UK, 16, 17, 30, 65, 143
uncertainty, 23, 27
uniform, 77
universe, 23, 31
urinary dysfunction, 116
urine, 48
users, 140
uterus, 134

V

validity, 68, 92
values, 23, 72
variability, 22, 26, 92
variable, 40, 70, 75, 87
variables, 36
variation, 40
vascular dementia, 106, 112, 115
vascular diseases, 122
vasodilation, 45
vasopressin, 43
venlafaxine, 118
ventilation, 63
ventricle, 79
Venus, 13
verbal aggressiveness, 106
vertebral artery, 82
victims, 131
violent crime, 131
violent crimes, 131
vision, 8, 24, 32, 83
visual area, 24
visual attention, 83
visual stimuli, 137
visualization, 3
vocabulary, 4, 13, 87, 113
vocalizations, 66, 69
voice, 6, 72

vulnerability, 122

W

waking, 2, 22, 32, 36, 37, 43, 44, 46, 55, 60, 73, 82
walking, 53, 54, 94
wavelengths, 8
weakness, 134
wealth, 3
Western countries, 49
white matter, 106, 115
William James, 145
windows, 77
winning, 11, 26
withdrawal, 47, 48, 49, 50, 70
witnesses, 96
women, 133, 134, 137
working memory, 27, 46, 81
World Trade Center, 130, 142
worldview, 8
writing, 5, 28

X

xerostomia, 48

Y

yes/no, 66, 67
yield, 29
young adults, 54

Z

ziprasidone, 118